STUDY
WITHOUT
STRESS

D1453815

This book is dedicated to all
students of the medical sciences.

EUGENIA G. KELMAN

KATHLEEN C. STRAKER

STUDY WITHOUT STRESS

Mastering Medical Sciences

Sage Publications, Inc.
International Educational and Professional Publisher
Thousand Oaks ▪ London ▪ New Delhi

For information:

Sage Publications, Inc.
2455 Teller Road
Thousand Oaks, California 91320
E-mail: order@sagepub.com

Sage Publications Ltd.
6 Bonhill Street
London EC2A 4PU
United Kingdom

Sage Publications India Pvt. Ltd.
M-32 Market
Greater Kailash I
New Delhi 110 048 India

Printed in the United States of America

ISBN 978-0-7619-1679-6

This book is printed on acid-free paper.

08 09 10 9 8 7 6 5

Acquiring Editor:	Jim Nageotte
Editorial Assistant:	Heidi Van Middlesworth
Production Editor:	Wendy Westgate
Editorial Assistant:	Nevair Kabakian
Copy Editor:	Linda Gray
Designer/Typesetter:	Janelle LeMaster
Cover Designer:	Ravi Balasuriya

Contents

Foreword

Few schools teach the most basic and essential skill for academic success: How to study. Most entering medical students discover that, although they earned good grades in college, they are not adequately prepared for the demanding pace and the overwhelming volume of material that needs to be learned.

Study Without Stress will help you take charge of your learning while greatly decreasing your stress. It provides a proven, effective way to balance your intellectual and emotional needs. Based on research literature and the authors' interactions with hundreds of students who participated in their workshops on study skills and stress management, *Study Without Stress* offers very specific and practical remedies to the unrelenting pressures inherent in medical school.

This book teaches how to manage your time, how to identify what is most important to learn, how to condense notes from the materials studied, how to review material efficiently and effectively, and how to test yourself to ensure that you know the material.

Kelman and Straker offered five- to six-week study skills workshops for interested students at the University of Texas Medical Branch, along with other more traditional tutorial programs. The medical school "grapevine" brought hundreds of students to these workshops over the years. The system consistently worked, because it allowed workshop participants to diagnose specific study skills deficiencies and showed them how to make corrections and incorporate these practical exercises into their daily schedules.

Other students who have also used the *Study Without Stress* program attest to its helpfulness, not only in establishing an effective, systematic approach to the information they must remember but also in thinking more rationally and calmly about the tasks before them.

No other single book combines these features or is specifically designed for the unique, intense learning environment of the medical sciences. *Study Without Stress* can be used by students in *any* educational setting or at any stage of learning.

Eugenia Kelman, Ph.D., and Kathleen Straker, M.Ed., have 25 years of combined experience in teaching study skills to medical and veterinary students. A counseling psychologist, Dr. Kelman became interested in developing academic support programs after discovering in her dissertation research that fear of academic failure was the major source of veterinary medical student stress. She later designed academic support programs for veterinary students at Cornell and Colorado State Universities and for allopathic medical students at the University of Texas Medical Branch. She has also conducted workshops on test anxiety desensitization and the control of stress through cognitive behavior management for undergraduate as well as medical students.

Kathleen Straker, an educator and reading specialist formerly in Student Affairs and Medical Education at the University of Texas Medical Branch, collaborated with Dr. Kelman in developing criterion-based instructional materials and offered study skills and reading enhancement workshops to medical students. She also served as Executive Chief Proctor for the National Board of Medical Examiners.

Medical students have consistently told the authors that if they had learned and used the *Study Without Stress* method during preprofessional preparation they would have had an easier time and earned much better grades. Everyone who has read a draft of this book has remarked, "I wish I had seen this book earlier; how can I get a copy?"

—Robert Holman Coombs
Professor of Behavioral Sciences, UCLA School of Medicine
Series Editor

Acknowledgments

We want to thank the students who attended our workshops over the years to learn how to study without stress. Not only were you receptive to our ideas, but you added to our understanding of what it takes to succeed in medical school by testing and refining the Study Without Stress system as you applied it to your own lives as medical students. Many of you also brought your best charts and diagrams to us and encouraged us to share them with others. We couldn't have written this book without you.

Special thanks to Kent Folsom M.D. and Jennifer Peel, Ph.D., for permission to reproduce some of their charts for this book and to Pat Ashford for using her computer graphics skills to translate those charts into this book's format. We also thank our reviewers for their helpful comments and suggestions, especially Janie Perez, R.N., M.A., P.N.P.

In addition, we would like to thank Dr. Robert H. Coombs, editor of the Surviving Medical School Series, and Dan Ruth, former Health Science Editor, and all those at Sage Publications who helped bring our book to fruition.

Introduction

Student (looking downcast):   "I just don't understand why I got a D on the Physiology midterm. I have a good general knowledge of physiology!"

Mentor: "Were there any general questions on the exam?"

Student (gazing off, considering):   "Well . . . no."

Learning in Medical School Is Different

Most students of medicine discover that, although they made good grades in college, they haven't developed adequate study skills for the volume and pace of material in medical school. Typically, this discovery is made either while preparing for the first exam or within moments of completing it. Usually, by the end of the first term—or at the latest, by the end of the first year—students stumble onto a workable system. This is crucial because the second year is even more intense. This book is for students who would like to avoid that scenario, take charge of their learning, and greatly decrease their stress, particularly in the first 2 years of medical school, whether in allopathic, dental, osteopathic, or veterinary medicine.

The immense volume of information to learn, the heavy emphasis on testing for detailed knowledge, and the apparent lack of time to accomplish even the minimum of what must be done all combine to make adjustment to the life of a medical student difficult. And stressful.

1

The typical premed student spends 35 to 40 hours a week in learning activities and is probably considered a "grind" by undergraduate peers not struggling to get into medical school. For undergraduate work, a careful reading of the required texts and acquiring a general idea of the content of the courses usually suffice to get a satisfactory grade. In contrast, medical students typically spend 60 to 65 hours a week in learning activities. A 1-hour medical school lecture may cover as much material as a premedical course covered in a week or more. "General" knowledge of the subject will not lead to the correct answers on detailed medical school exams. Most exams require specific knowledge and often ask for application of that knowledge to solve a problem.

Thus, during their first year of medical school, students must

- learn to lead highly disciplined lives, postpone ordinary pleasures, and devote much more time to work than other people they know;
- become excellent time managers, to squeeze in enough time for basic human needs, such as eating, sleeping, and exercise; and
- figure out how to connect and retain an enormous amount of information.

Course material is presented so rapidly that it often seems impossible to keep Monday's lecture and laboratory content safely filed away in the brain until Friday, never mind that a similar number of facts, which must also be remembered, will be added every day in between. No wonder medical students dream of having total recall, invent mnemonic devices, and buy lots of books and tapes about memory improvement!

Cramming Doesn't Make Good Use of Time

Although "pulling an all-nighter" might have saved the grade in a premedical course, cramming is not functional in medical school and is usually associated with lower academic achievement and higher stress. If it takes between 60 to 65 hours a week to cover the volume of material and the student distributes those hours unevenly, concentrating them just prior to a test, a pattern of time usage between tests emerges, as shown in Figure 0.1.

The debt of study time accumulated early in the period between exams must be paid in the week or two immediately before the test. The interest on this debt of time is fatigue, vulnerability to illness due to lack of sleep and poor eating habits, the temptation to use "uppers" to keep awake and alert before and during the exam, and chronic anxiety. When they are not working up to speed, "crammers" inwardly chide themselves and worry about what they are

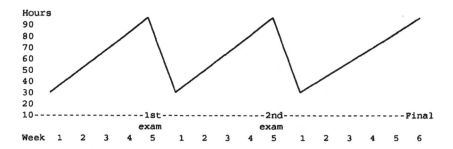

Figure 0.1. Student Who "Crams"

NOTE: This "crammer" averages 60 to 65 hours of study per week during the intertest period but earns more stress and learns less than the student who consistently keeps a 60- to 65-hour schedule of study.

not doing, knowing they will have to pay for their inactivity; as the test approaches, they are prey to anxious thoughts about the difficulty of the task of getting all that information into memory at once and about possible failure. The stress increases proportionally to the increase in the workload as the next exam approaches and then peaks in the days just prior to a test. They feel "stressed out" and describe themselves as "living from test to test."

The student who follows the Study Without Stress (SWS) system will work at a steady pace between exams (see Figure 0.2).

Cramming Doesn't Promote Long-Term Memory

Psychologists have researched learning, memory, and retention for over 100 years. It's hard to distinguish between learning and memory because the only way to measure what you know is to ask you either to recall it or use it in solving a problem. Learning is memory, in the sense that what is remembered is what has been learned. Retention is the ability to retrieve what has been learned in the past. Scientists have not found a biological basis for the limitation of learning. Apparently, whatever has been learned in the past, after infancy, continues to exist in the brain. The problem is **retrieval.** We've all stared at a test question and thought, "I know that. I can even vaguely see in my mind's eye the page in the book where I read it. I just can't bring it into focus and come up with the particular fact needed to answer this question!" The ability to retrieve is the only test of learning, however. The first 2 years of medical school seem to be an endless series of those tests.

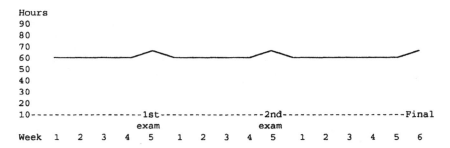

Figure 0.2. Student Who Is on a Steady Schedule

NOTE: Maintaining a relatively steady rate of 60 to 65 hours of study time per week costs exactly the same amount of time as cramming but avoids the final period of panic to which "crammers" subject themselves. This stable pattern also permits a review of previously studied material. The small rise just before exams in the steady-state study pattern is for extra review.

Keys to Memory

Scientists who have studied learning and retention have identified the following factors as keys to memory:

- *Organization* of the facts into logical patterns means that information can be learned initially and retained for a longer period of time. This is one of the "hottest" and most productive areas in research on learning and retention.

- *Distributed practice* (review at regular intervals) results in more learning and retention than massed practice (one intense period of study), commonly known as "cramming."

- *Repetition* increases learning and retention and retards "forgetting" (failure to retrieve). There are many examples of this in everyday life. Tying shoelaces, for example, is done without any apparent cognitive effort because we've repeated the task so often, but it is actually a rather complicated maneuver.

- The *amount of time* from the learning experience until the time of recall or recognition makes a difference. More than a century ago, Ebbinghaus plotted the "Curve of Forgetting" (see Figure 0.3), which describes the amount of information that is "lost" (cannot be retrieved) over time elapsed since the initial "learning."

- *Intent to remember* includes mental rehearsal, effort, use of clear imagery, a positive suggestion, and your attitude toward the subject or value attached to the subject.

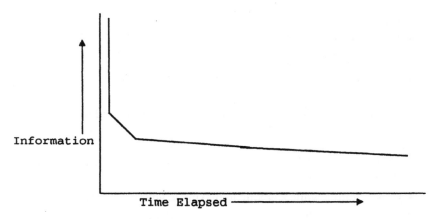

Figure 0.3. Forgetting Curve

NOTE: Published in 1885, Ebbinghaus demonstrated how information is forgotten with the passage of time, unless the information is brought to mind (reviewed) on a regular basis.

- *Varied input modality* strengthens learning, perhaps because the information received in different ways (visual, auditory, kinesthetic) is stored differently in the brain. Use of varied modalities uses all capacities of the brain and optimizes neural interchange (theoretically). Use all the learning tools possible!

Mnemonic devices help in short-term memory—for example, remembering names of people you meet at a party—but probably are of little use in retention of medical science. Medical students sometimes buy "Improving Your Memory" books in the hope that the mnemonic suggestions will help them on their tests, but typically they don't. The great quantity of material to be stored and the fact that you must first learn or invent the mnemonic and its proper associations actually make learning mnemonic devices an inefficient use of time.

Overview of the Study Without Stress System

The SWS system puts scientific principles of learning and retention into practice for medical students and students in any other similarly challenging curricula. For any unit of study (topic, chapter) there are four distinct steps. These are covered in sequential order:

- Prereading
- Note making
- Reviewing
- Self-testing

To assist you in executing each of these steps, we offer additional chapters devoted to the following:

- Managing your schedule to guarantee enough time for each of the four steps
- Concentrating while studying to maximize your use of time
- Taking tests skillfully to use all your knowledge
- Overcoming the anxiety of taking tests

If repetition and conceptual organization of the information are important for retention, *time* must first be scheduled for creating organized notes that can be reviewed repeatedly. Time is the essential foundation. The first chapter is designed, therefore, to ensure that you are steadily scheduling, on a weekly basis, an adequate amount of time for note making and review. It is nearly impossible to have repeated practice (review) without a highly organized set of condensed notes. The chapter on *reading and note making* teaches how to create a set of highly organized, condensed notes that relate the details to the general concepts you are studying. Recent research indicates that looking for connections and relationships in material leads to greater comprehension and retention. We even tell you in the chapter on *reviewing and self-testing* how to be sure you know what you think you know before the test. (It's less fun to find out during the test.)

The chapters on *prereading and concentration* will help you get the most out of your 60-plus hours a week. If you are more efficient in using the hours you schedule, you have the choice of either increasing your detailed knowledge or having more available time for other activities. Students who faithfully follow the recommendations in these chapters say that their learning productivity per hour increases as much as 20%.

The chapter on *test taking* is designed to give you an overview of the types of objective test items most commonly used in medical schools and on board examinations. Also included are tips on how to "work" test items in a way that will fully use all the information you have filed away.

Dealing with *test-taking anxiety* is a final supplement to the SWS method. This chapter will help you avoid the distractions of physical and emotional

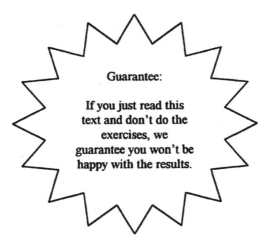

Guarantee:

If you just read this
text and don't do the
exercises, we
guarantee you won't be
happy with the results.

tension while preparing for tests and while taking them. You will then be able to concentrate your energy on retrieving your stored information and using your good test-taking strategies. Many of the suggestions in this chapter are useful when you're not taking tests, too.

SWS is interactive. This book is not just for reading. You will get out of this only what you put into it, so we urge you to do the exercises! The authors have used these methods in workshops with hundreds of veterinary and allopathic medical students for many years. Didactic material is kept to a minimum. Exercises are emphasized with the thought that you will learn and retain more from actions than words. By completing the exercises, you will be more likely to integrate this new learning into your future behavior. We want you to teach yourself the best way to learn—through active practice.

How to Use This Book

The best way to use this book is to progress according to the following timeline:

Week 1   Read and do exercises in Chapters 1 and 2.

Week 2   Read and do exercises in Chapter 3 while continuing exercises for Chapters 1 and 2.

Week 3   Read and add exercises in Chapter 4 to the preceding chapters.

Week 4   Read and do exercises in Chapter 5, while continuing study components introduced in Chapters 1 through 4.

Week 5   Read and do exercises in Chapter 6. By this week, all basic study
          elements should be integrated into your overall study plan.

Week 6   If you have a problem with test-taking anxiety, read and do
          exercises in Chapter 7.

Structure of the Chapters

Chapters include the following elements:

- *Diagnostic exercise.* You will diagnose yourself by describing your
  current approach to the chapter topic. An annotated scoring guide will
  help you decide how much of the content applies to you.
- *Background on the topic* and why it is important for medical students.
- *Exercises for active practice.* Specific activities to improve your performance are prescribed, sometimes with worksheets provided to record
  your efforts.
- *Exercise for evaluation.* What did you learn? How will that knowledge
  change the way you study in the future?
- *"Students Say."* In their own words, students who have participated in
  our workshops reflect on how the chapter topic affected their work.
- *Summary of main points.*
- *Review of literature.* For those who want to know more, we have supplied
  an annotated set of references.

If You Want to Know More

Arnold, L., & Feighney, K. M. (1995). Students' general learning approaches and
    performances in medical school: A longitudinal study. *Academic Medicine,
    70*(8), 715-725.

> *Students who depend on rote memorizing and a fragmented approach to
> learning have reduced performance over 6 years of medical education and
> training. Those who look for connections and relationships in material have
> higher achievement. Authors argue against mnemonic devices and a memo-
> rizing approach.*

Boring, E. G., Langfeld, H. S., & Weld, H. P. (1948). *Foundations of psychology.* New York: John Wiley.

Chapter 8 deals with retention and transfer of learning.

Coles, C. R. (1990). Helping students with learning difficulties in medical and health care education. *Medical Education, 24,* 300-312.

Medical students experiencing difficulty in studying report the following problems: not organizing study time efficiently; feeling overwhelmed, over-loaded, and overworked; losing their initial motivation; becoming more cynical and pessimistic; questioning the necessity of their coursework; becoming anxious and questioning whether they belong in medical school.

Colvin, R. H., & Taylor, D. D. (1978). Planning student work-study time in an objectives-based medical curriculum. *Journal of Medical Education, 53,* 393-396.

The authors calculate that a final review, "cramming," takes 1 hour for every 10 hours of reading and review.

Ebbinghaus, H. (1885). *Über das Gedächtnis.* Leipzig, Germany: Dunker & Humbolt.

Describes how we forget over time.

Farr, M. J. (1987). *The long-term retention of knowledge and skills.* New York: Springer-Verlag.

A thorough review of the scientific literature on learning, memory, and retention, including the Ebbinghaus work originally published in 1885.

Jacobson, R. L. (1986, September 3). Memory experts' advice: Forget about that string around your finger. *Chronicle of Higher Education,* p. 49.

A survey of 68 psychologists actively involved in research on memory revealed their personal preference for writing things down as an aid to retention. In addition, they prefer organization and repetition. They do not recommend the use of mnemonic devices for most practical applications.

Kelman, E. G. (1978). Stressors for veterinary medical students and types of students reporting most stress. *Journal of Veterinary Medical Education, 5*(3), 145-151.

Fear of failure and limited time to absorb a vast quantity of information leads 20% to 30% of students to seek some form of counseling. Principal stressors reported by students are tests and lack of time.

Polk, S. R. (1995). *The medical student's survival guide: Career strategy for changing times.* Myrtle Beach, SC: Trentland.

Stress in basic sciences years stems from study schedules made overly harsh by inefficient study techniques.

Sisson, J. C., Swartz, R. D., & Wolf, F. M. (1992). Learning, retention and recall of clinical information. *Medical Education, 26,* 454-461.

Thirty-three medical students lost between 10% and 20% comprehension when taking the same test 3 months later with no review.

Spitzer, H. F. (1939). Studies in retention. *Journal of Educational Psychology, 30,* 641-656.

Study of forgetting before and after review shows significantly greater retention up to 60 days after reading, if material is reviewed. Concludes review should occupy 90% to 95% of study time, especially if material is somewhat disconnected or detailed.

1 Time
Your Greatest Resource

(Weeks 1 and 2)

Student: All I ever do is study, but I'm not making the grades I need.

Mentor: So, how much time do you study?

Student: I don't know. It seems like all the time.

Before reading this chapter, take a few minutes for a diagnosis:

Diagnose Yourself: How Do You Use Your Time Now?

Directions: Circle the number that best describes your actual behavior during an academic term.

Never
Rarely
Sometimes
Often
Always

0 1 2 3 4   1. I keep a daily schedule or personal calendar of appointments and high-priority tasks.

0 1 2 3 4   2. I schedule some time (one hour) for fun or physical exercise every day (or several times a week).

4 3 2 1 0   3. I take a few days off from studying right after in-term examinations.

4 3 2 1 0   4. I have no time to sleep just before examinations and therefore feel very tired during exams.

0 1 2 3 4   5. I make a point of getting 50 minutes of concentrated study for every hour of scheduled study time.

0 1 2 3 4   6. I carry a personal calendar or schedule as a handy reference.

4 3 2 1 0   7. I find it necessary to make excuses or apologize for being late, missing appointments, or arriving at the wrong time or place for an appointment.

0 1 2 3 4   8. I get enough sleep so as not to feel sleepy during the day.

0 1 2 3 4   9. I know fairly accurately how much time is spent on various activities on a daily and weekly basis.

4 3 2 1 0   10. I allow calls or visits from friends to interfere with following a study schedule.

0 1 2 3 4   11. I have designated times to carry out daily and weekly tasks.

0 1 2 3 4   12. I consult a personal calendar or schedule each day.

0 1 2 3 4   13. I say "no" to invitations that irretrievably interfere with a planned study schedule.

0 1 2 3 4   14. I check a personal calendar or schedule before agreeing to take on a project or attend an activity.

0 1 2 3 4   15. I carry something to study while waiting for class to begin, between classes, waiting to meet a friend, and the like.

4 3 2 1 0   16. I postpone studying to accept a social invitation during a scheduled study time.

4 3 2 1 0   17. I study only when "in the mood."

4 3 2 1 0   18. I plan to do most personal studying (as differentiated from lecture and labs) on the weekends.

4 3 2 1 0   19. I fall asleep while studying.

4 3 2 1 0   20. I watch television more than one hour per day.

__68__   **Total score** (sum of circled items)

21. Estimate how much time you spend on pleasurable activities/recreation (not including deliberate physical exercise) on a weekly basis.   _25_ hours per week

22. Estimate how much time you spend on deliberate physical exercise on a weekly basis.   _4_ hours per week

23. About how much time do you spend attending lectures and labs on a weekly basis?   _20_ hours per week

24. Approximately how much time do you spend in personal study (i.e., studying on your own, not in lecture or lab) on a weekly basis?   _32_ hours per week

7p-12a

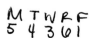

M T W R F
5 4 3 6 1

25 M-F + 6 — 32hr

25. About how much time do you spend on housekeeping, shopping, personal hygiene, and eating
per week?   **21** hours per week

26. On the average, how many hours do you sleep
per night?   **6** hours per night

☞ Stop.
Do not continue until you are
ready to score the Time-Use Inventory.

Scoring Directions: Time Management Diagnosis

Add up all your answers on Items 1 through 20. Your score is the
total of the numbers you circled.   **68**

1. Keeping a daily schedule or personal calendar for appointments and
high-priority tasks saves brain cells to remember information you need
to recall on tests. Why distract yourself with mental "to do" lists or
scheduled appointments when you can refer to a written record and check
them off as they are completed? ✓

2. Everyone deserves an hour of fun a day, or life gets pretty dull. Because
being a medical student requires so much sitting, the more physically
active your recreation, the better! ✓

3. It is not a good idea to take a few days off from studying right after an
exam, because then you have to play "catch up," which is extremely
draining, thus creating the vicious cycle of procrastination: panic—
cramming—procrastination (wanting to rest), and so on. ✓

4. Careful planning of the period between exams will allow you time for
review *and* sleep, which will probably help your test performance. Not
getting enough sleep just before exams is diagnostic of cramming. ✓

5. If you make a point of getting 50 minutes of concentrated study for every
hour of scheduled study time, you will be using your time more efficiently
and you may not even need to put in as many hours! ✓

6. If you carry a personal calendar or schedule with you (and consult it
daily), you will have a more accurate gauge of your time commitments,
which will allow you to make better decisions concerning your time. Also,
see Number 1 about saving brain space whenever possible by carrying
written reminders.

7. If you find it necessary to make excuses or apologies about not keeping appointments, you probably are not recording (and consulting daily) your schedule of appointments and "to do" list.

8. Not getting enough sleep is like deficit spending: You end up paying it back with interest. Better to stick to a sensible schedule allowing at least seven hours sleep a night and really be awake and alert when you study.

9. Having an accurate estimate of time usage is the first step toward spending it more efficiently.

10. Sticking to a study schedule ensures that you spend the time needed to accomplish your goals, and then you are able to spend "guilt-free" time enjoying yourself. If you allow others to change your schedule on a routine basis, you've lost control of deciding what you want to do with your limited time for recreational activities.

11. See Number 10.

12. Consulting your personal calendar or schedule at the beginning of each day (and throughout the day) ensures that you will remember what you'd planned to do. See Numbers 1, 6, and 7 above.

13. See Number 10. It is not an "irretrievable" loss of study time if you can swap a recreational period elsewhere that same week and make up the study time.

14. Checking your calendar or schedule before agreeing to take on a project or attend an activity helps you stick to your planned schedule and prevents the unpleasant social chore of later "backing out" of engagements.

15. Get into the habit of carrying something to study during those odd bits of time. You will free up other bits of time because of the studying you have accomplished in time otherwise lost during the day.

16. See Number 10.

17. When you are a doctor, you will not have the luxury of going to work only when you feel like it. Better to learn now to "act yourself into feeling"—to do it even if you don't feel like it.

18. Planning to do most of your personal studying on the weekends will not allow you to keep current with the material, especially if some urgent event requires more of your time than planned.

19. Falling asleep while studying is not a good study habit or an efficient use of time. Try to plan your studying during a "peak" energy time in your day. Anyway, it's more comfortable to sleep in bed than on top of your books and notes.

20. Watching television more than one hour per day indicates poor time management. Ask yourself, "Is seeing another rerun of *Star Trek* really worth the anxious cramming I'll have to do before the next exam?"

Score Interpretation: Time Management Diagnosis

If your score on the first 20 items is in the **60-80** range, you could skip this chapter. You're a good time manager. However, if you want to feel smug and superior, you might read it just for fun.

If your score is in the **40-59** range, you have the basic concepts but need practice and perseverance. Do the exercises in this chapter to reinforce your best behavior.

If your score was **below 40,** read on! This chapter may be the solution to your main problem. Time is the essential building block of all the other skills prescribed in this book. You simply cannot succeed without allocating sufficient time to learning activities.

A Day in the Life of a Student

The alarm rings at 7:30 a.m. and Student jumps out of bed, takes a quick shower, digs through the pile of clothes on the floor, throws on what he hopes is a clean pair of underwear, and grabs a cup of coffee. He gets to his 8:00 class at 8:05 and slips into an empty seat in the back of the lecture hall. He props his eyelids open for the next two hours of lectures. He's too hungry to sit through the 10:00 class and goes to the cafeteria to get a bagel and a cup of coffee. He returns for the 11:00 lecture feeling more awake. He has lunch with his friends, and they bemoan the fact that there's never time for anything but studying. He has lab most of the afternoon. At 4:00 p.m., he goes to the gym to work out. An hour and a half later, he's on his way home to clean up for dinner. Dinner at his medical fraternity is at 6:00. Student and his friends discuss how there isn't enough time to do all the studying that needs to be done. At 7:00 p.m., he gets ready to study. He picks up his biochemistry book and starts reading the assigned chapters. At 7:30 he remembers he has an anatomy lab tomorrow and picks up his lab manual. Fifteen minutes later, the phone rings. When he hangs up at 8:15, he's forgotten what he was studying, so he rereads part of the lab manual. By 8:30, he needs a break and heads to the kitchen to get a snack and shoot the breeze with a friend. At 9:00, he decides to finish that biochemistry chapter, even though he hasn't finished preparing for lab. He begins to tire of reading at 9:30 and decides to take a TV break. He goes back to reading at 10:30 p.m. and has trouble understanding the Krebs cycle. His eyes begin shutting involuntarily, and at 11:00 he decides to get ready for bed and takes his books with him to bed. By 11:30, he's drifted off clutching his biochemistry book to his chest, snoring gently.

The next day when his parents call and ask what he's been doing, he says, "Are you kidding? I don't do anything but study!"

Realistically, how much did Student study during his typical day? Although he sat in lecture for three hours, he missed more than half of the content because he wasn't prepared. He had three hours of lab, for which he was also not prepared. If you count up the actual time he spent in personal study, it comes to only about two hours. Although it seemed that the day was filled with nothing but study, Student Doctor spent less than the average amount of time in personal study that medical students need to succeed. Never mind at this point whether any of his study was quality time!

How Students of Medicine Spend Their Time

Research indicates that medical and veterinary medical students spend between 60 and 65 hours per week in learning tasks (classes, labs, and personal study). *Is* there that much time? Let's take a look at how much time is available in a week.

We all have exactly 168 hours (7 days × 24 hours) to spend every week.

The typical medical student reports **sleeping** about 7 to 7.5 hours a night (except before a big exam).	168 −51 ———
That leaves you 117 hours for everything else.	117
Most medical schools schedule about 30 hours per week in **organized study activities** (i.e., lectures, labs, recitations) during basic science years.	117 −30 —— 87
Studies of time use by medical students suggest that they spend 30 to 35 hours per week in **personal study,** varying according to the quality of their premedical preparation for the curriculum.	87 −35 —— 52
You can't live without eating, and most students say they spend about 2 hours a day preparing **meals**, eating, and cleaning afterward.	52 −14 —— 38

Now that you've slept, gone to class, studied, and eaten, you have   38
38 hours left.

Although people vary in how much time they want to spend on   38
maintenance activities (housekeeping, laundry, shopping, minor   −7
repairs, etc.), a reasonable average would probably be about 7   31
hours a week.

Personal hygiene is another use of time that varies greatly among   31
individuals, but our experience is that a student can keep reason-   −7
ably clean and neat (showering, shaving, hair care, dressing, etc.)   24
at the rate of about an hour a day.

This leaves 24 hours every week for rest and recreation (R&R)! A well-organized student could use 3 hours every weekday for R&R and still have an additional 9 hours free on the weekend.

If you have to commute any great distance or have familial or parental obligations, however, those duties will have to come out of this remaining 24 hours (and there won't be much left).

If you ask Student Doctor if he had any time free for R&R during that typical day we recounted earlier, he might acknowledge the hour at the gym and the hour in front of the TV. The other time just slipped through his fingers. At the end of the day, he didn't feel he'd accomplished as much as he should.

Where did those hours go? Read on to find out . . .

Exercise 1: Measure How You Presently Use Your Time

The first step in planning efficient use of time is to analyze what you actually do with your time *now*. Do not let the fear that you will discover you waste time keep you from doing this important exercise. The odds are high that you waste a couple of hours every day. Accept that as a possible fact and do an honest tally of what you *really* do with your time now.

Remove the Baseline Time-Monitoring form (Table 1.1). You can make extra copies of it before marking on it, in case you need more forms later. Carry one with you for the next seven days. If you like, you can fill in all your scheduled and unalterable activities first (lectures, labs, meetings or work obligations, commute time, worship, and any special appointments or dates to which you are already committed).

Write in the boxes for each hour or half-hour everything you do according to the following categories:

- Lecture (LEC)
- Laboratory (LAB)
- Scheduled learning activities (SLA) (seminars, tutorials, review sessions)
- Personal study (PS)
- Maintenance (M)—includes a wide variety of "have to do" tasks, such as housecleaning, taking care of your car, laundry, cooking, eating, and shopping (for food and other essentials, not wandering the mall, which would be considered R&R)
- Sleeping (S)
- Physical exercise (PE)
- Employed hours (JOB)

Count anything that doesn't fit in these categories (including parental duties or commuting) as R&R, ridiculous as that may seem. Later, you can create your own form or use a scheduling book that you can customize.

Here's how two different students recorded their baseline time usage (see Tables 1.2 and 1.3).

Linda R. did her baseline monitoring exercise during the fall term of her first year of medical school. As you will see, she is short on personal study time because of her commute, familial obligations, and maintaining her home and yard. She is an older married student with a child. Linda has very little R&R and almost no physical exercise. She's always busy but does not arrange enough personal study to keep up with her classes.

Kenneth B. completed the baseline during spring semester of his first year. He had approximately the same number of scheduled classes and labs as Linda but no commute and average maintenance activities. He is a single young man living in student housing where his meals are provided. Kenneth had enough personal study time on the weekdays, but apparently he thought that was enough and left the weekends for total R&R. This is unrealistic. If he added eight hours of weekend personal study time, which is more typical of a well-organized medical student, he would be in the average range. Kenneth needs to cut down on R&R.

From the baseline time-monitoring exercise, both Linda and Kenneth learned that they needed to change their lifestyles to allow more time for personal study. Linda decided to make better use of her commute time by listening to audiotaped lectures and study notes while driving, make better use of her time on campus between classes, and try to cut down or delegate some

Table 1.1 Time-Monitoring Form

Record your activities in one hour or in half-hour units for one week. At the end of the week, calculate totals for major activities using the following categories: LEC (lecture), LAB (laboratory), SLA (scheduled learning activities—e.g., seminars, review sessions), PS (personal study), JOB (employed hours), M (maintenance activities—shopping, cooking, cleaning, errands, eating, personal hygiene, etc.), PE (physical exercise), S (sleep), R&R (rest and recreation—anything that does not fit into previous categories).

Name _____ Week of _____

	Monday	Tuesday	Wednesday	Thursday	Friday	Saturday
5:30 a						
6:00						
6:30						
7:00						
7:30						
8:00						
9:00						
10:00						
11:00						
12:00						
12:30 p						
1:00						
2:00						
3:00						
4:00						
5:00						
5:30						
6:00						
6:30						
7:00						
7:30						
8:00						
8:30						
9:00						
9:30						
10:00						
10:30						
11:00						
11:30						
12:00						
12:30 a						
1:00						
1:30						
2:00						

Daily totals

	Monday	Tuesday	Wednesday	Thursday	Friday	Saturday
All study						
Main						
PE						
R&R						
Sleep						

Weekly totals: Study = ____; Main = ____; PE = ____; Sleep = ____

Table 1.2   Linda R.'s Time-Monitoring Schedule

Record your activities in one hour or in half-hour units for one week. At the end of the week, calculate totals for major activities using the following categories: LEC (lecture), LAB (laboratory), SLA (scheduled learning activities—e.g., seminars, review sessions), PS (personal study), JOB (employed hours), M (maintenance activities—shopping, cooking, cleaning, errands, eating, personal hygiene, etc.), PE (physical exercise), S (sleep), R&R (rest and recreation—anything that does not fit into previous categories).

Name _____ *Linda R.* _____ Week of ___*October 18-25*___

	Monday	Tuesday	Wednesday	Thursday	Friday	Saturday	Sunday
5:30 a	Sleep	Sleep	Sleep	Sleep	Sleep	Sleep	Sleep
6:00	Main	M	M	M	S	S	S
6:30	M	M	M	M	M	S	S
7:00	(commute)	(commute)	(commute)	(commute)	(commute)	M	S
7:30	M	M	M	M	M	M	S
8:00	LEC	LEC	PS	LEC	LEC	M	M
9:00	LEC	LEC	LEC	LEC	LEC	PS	M
10:00	LAB	LAB	R&R	LAB	PS	PS	M
11:00	LAB	LAB	LEC	LAB	M	PS	M
12:00	M	M	M	M	M	M	M
12:30 p	M	M	M	M	M	M	M
1:00	LEC	LEC	LEC	LEC	LEC	M	R&R
2:00	LAB	M	LAB	LEC	LAB	M	R&R
3:00	LAB	PS	LAB	M	LAB	R&R	M
4:00	PS	SLA	LAB	M	LAB	R&R	M
5:00	M	M	M	M	LAB	R&R	M
5:30	M	M	M	M	M	M	M
6:00	M	M	M	M	M	M	M
6:30	M	M	M	R&R	M	M	M
7:00	PS	M	R&R	R&R	M	M	PS
7:30	PS	PS	R&R	M	R&R	PS	PS
8:00	PS	PS	R&R	PS	R&R	PS	PS
8:30	M	PS	M	M	R&R	M	M
9:00	PS	PS	R&R	PS	R&R	PS	R&R
9:30	PS	PS	R&R	PS	R&R	PS	PS
10:00	PS	PS	PS	PS	R&R	R&R	PS
10:30	R&R	R&R	PS	PS	R&R	R&R	PS
11:00	M	R&R	PS	M	PS	S	M
11:30	Sleep	M	Sleep	Sleep	M		S
12:00		Sleep			Sleep		
12:30 a							

Daily totals

All study	10.5	10	7	8.5	8.5	5	3
Main	6	7	5.5	8	6	7.5	12.5
PE	0	0	0	0	0	0	0
R&R	.5	1	2.5	1	3.5	3	2.5
Sleep	6.5	6	6.5	7	7	9	6.5

Weekly totals: Study = <u>52.5</u>; Main = <u>34</u>; PE = <u>0</u>; R&R = <u>14</u>; Sleep = <u>48.5</u>

Table 1.3   Kenneth B.'s Time-Monitoring Schedule

Record your activities in one hour or in half-hour units for one week. At the end of the week, calculate totals for major activities using the following categories: LEC (lecture), LAB (laboratory), SLA (scheduled learning activities—e.g., seminars, review sessions), PS (personal study), JOB (employed hours), M (maintenance activities—shopping, cooking, cleaning, errands, eating, personal hygiene, etc.), PE (physical exercise), S (sleep), R&R (rest and recreation—anything that does not fit into previous categories).

Name _____ *Kenneth B.* _____   Week of ___ *January 17-23* ___

	Monday	Tuesday	Wednesday	Thursday	Friday	Saturday	Sunday
5:30 a	Sleep	Sleep	Sleep	Sleep	Sleep	Sleep	Sleep
6:00	S	S	S	S	S	S	S
6:30	S	S	S	S	S	S	S
7:00	M	M	M	M	M	S	S
7:30	M	M	M	M	M	S	S
8:00	LEC	LEC	PS	LEC	LEC	M	M
9:00	LEC	LEC	LEC	LEC	LEC	R&R	M
10:00	LAB	LEC	LEC	LAB	LAB	R&R	M
11:00	LAB	PS	LEC	LAB	LAB	R&R	R&R
12:00	M	M	M	M	M	R&R	R&R
12:30 p	PS	M	M	M	PS	R&R	R&R
1:00	IFL LAB	M	PS	PS	PS	M	R&R
2:00	LAB	LAB	PS	LAB	PS	R&R	R&R
3:00	LAB	LAB	PS	LAB	PS	PE	R&R
4:00	LAB	PS	SLA	PS	PE	PE	R&R
5:00	M	PS	M	M	PE	R&R	R&R
5:30	R&R	M	R&R	M	M	R&R	R&R
6:00	PS	M	PS	SLA	M	R&R	M
6:30	PS	R&R	PS	SLA	PS	M	M
7:00	PS	R&R	PS	M	PS	M	R&R
7:30	PS	PE	PS	PS	PS	R&R	R&R
8:00	PS	PE	PS	PS	PS	R&R	R&R
8:30	PS	PE	M	PS	PS	R&R	R&R
9:00	PS	PE	R&R	PS	R&R	R&R	R&R
9:30	PS	PS	R&R	R&R	R&R	R&R	R&R
10:00	R&R	PS	R&R	R&R	R&R	R&R	R&R
10:30	R&R	PS	R&R	R&R	R&R	R&R	R&R
11:00	R&R	R&R	R&R	R&R	R&R	R&R	R&R
11:30	M	R&R	R&R	R&R	R&R	R&R	R&R
12:00	Sleep	M	Sleep	Sleep	Sleep	R&R	R&R
12:30 a		Sleep				R&R	Sleep

Daily totals

All study	12.5	9.5	9.5	10	10	0	0
Main	2.5	4.5	3	3.5	2.5	3	4
PE	0	2	0	0	2	2	0
R&R	2	2	3.5	2.5	3	12.5	13
Sleep	7	6.5	7	7	7	7	7.5

Weekly totals: Study = <u>53.5</u>; Main = <u>23</u>; PE = <u>6</u>; R&R = <u>40.5</u>; Sleep = <u>49</u>

maintenance activities. Kenneth decided to forgo some of his weekend R&R when he planned his schedule for the next week.

Notice how different is the use of their nonscheduled time. Students who are married, have children, commute to school, or have part-time jobs will have very different lifestyles than do students who are single, live near school, and are not employed.

Always remember this rule when scheduling or monitoring study time: **Do not count any hour of personal study unless you actually study at least 50 minutes of that hour.**

Taking a 10-minute break between two hours of intensive study is OK, but if you take a break after 40 minutes, you cannot count it as an hour. Just to keep your schedule less cluttered looking, it's best not to schedule anything in less than half-hour periods (one-hour periods are more efficient, when you consider the time it takes to get started studying). If you do plan a half-hour study period, you must study 25 minutes of that time to count it as a half-hour of study.

Around meal times, the time-monitoring form is broken into half-hour units, because many students take about a half-hour for meals.

Use the time-monitoring sheet and begin **today** to collect baseline data on how you use your time. At the end of the baseline time-monitoring week, return to this chapter and complete "Check-Up for Exercise 1: Time Monitoring," to continue your time management program.

While you are doing this time-monitoring exercise for a week, skip forward to the next chapter. We urge, however, that you not go past the prereading chapter in this week. SWS is a step-by-step program. Stick to the suggested weekly schedule: Too much change all at once can be overwhelming. You'll find it is easy to incorporate one or two steps at a time as suggested.

☞ Go to Chapter 2, "Prereading."

Check-Up for Exercise 1: Time Monitoring

To be completed after monitoring your time for one week.

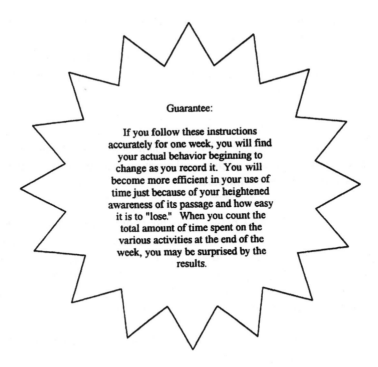

Guarantee:

If you follow these instructions accurately for one week, you will find your actual behavior beginning to change as you record it. You will become more efficient in your use of time just because of your heightened awareness of its passage and how easy it is to "lose." When you count the total amount of time spent on the various activities at the end of the week, you may be surprised by the results.

1. What did you learn from the time-monitoring exercise? (Write your response in the space provided.)

_____

_____

_____

2. How many hours did you actually spend per day in all learning activities (including lectures, labs, and personal study) during the time-monitoring period? There are places on your time-monitoring sheet to record daily and weekly totals, for all forms of study. Where is your total in comparison with the 60- to 65-hour per week average?

_____

_____

_____

Referring to your completed one-week baseline time-monitoring schedule, answer the following questions.

3. How much time do you actually spend on pleasurable activities/recreation (not including deliberate physical exercise) on a weekly basis? (R&R) _____ hours per week

4. How much time do you actually spend on deliberate physical exercise on a weekly basis? (PE) _____ hours per week

5. How much time do you actually spend attending lectures and labs on a weekly basis? (LEC, LAB) _____ hours per week

6. How much time do you actually spend in personal study (i.e., studying on your own, not in lecture or lab) on a weekly basis? (PS) _____ hours per week

7. How much time do you actually spend on maintenance activities, personal hygiene, and eating per week? (M) _____ hours per week

8. How many hours do you sleep per night? _____ hours per night

9. How close was your estimate of time allocation (at the beginning of this chapter) to the totals actually observed on your time-monitoring sheet?

_____

_____

_____

10. What do you need to change about your time management (highest priority)?

_____

_____

_____

11. What else do you need to change about your use of time (second-highest priority)?

_____

_____

_____

What Students Learn From This Exercise

Ways to waste time vary considerably among students. After completing the time-monitoring exercise for one week, one woman discovered that she was spending 21 hours a week on personal hygiene. She wasn't satisfied with her achievement as a medical student, because she was not giving her studies enough time to do them justice. She immediately cut the time spent on grooming by half.

Another student had to confront the fact that he was sleeping too much. Whenever he felt anxious or worried, he just took a nap to escape his unpleasant thoughts. He was sleeping about 10 hours a day. He thus avoided anxiety temporarily, but the 2 or 3 hours of lost study time every day only created more problems for him in the long run and made him even more anxious.

The most common finding of students who complete this exercise is, curiously, that they don't really enjoy the time they spend on R&R. Although their hourly tally of R&R time may have been high, there was no interesting activity during that time. Time that just slips away, like water through the fingers, has to be counted as R&R, if it doesn't fit into any other category. It can add up to a lot of time over a week. Scheduling enough time to engage in two or three really enjoyable activities that provide a refreshing break from all the tasks is a must. To keep work time separate from play and to have worthwhile recreational activities, it's better to schedule time for R&R and then really enjoy it. Once you have a schedule that's working for you, you can play with a guilt-free conscience, knowing your studies will be completed in the time you've scheduled for them.

Now are you motivated to use your time more efficiently next week? If so, read on . . .

Planning Your Schedule

Decide what is your best study time (this may be revised after you do the exercises in the chapter on concentration). By "best study time," we do not mean when you're in the mood but, rather, when you have a serious block of time (best if it's 2 or 3 hours in a sequence) to devote to study. Schedule such a block of time for personal study time every day. To do this, you must decide how long you can sustain a high level of concentration. By making a plan to study for at least three consecutive hours, you may be able to extend your period of concentration. If not, you'll want to schedule a break for R&R or a maintenance activity between periods of concentrated study. Maintenance activities, physical exercise, and R&R should be planned for time when you feel less mentally energetic or need a break from an intense period of study.

You should continue to count any hour as an hour of study if, and only if, you actually study 50 minutes of that hour. This will alert you to avoiding unplanned interruptions.

Whenever possible, plan a study period immediately after lecture to consolidate your notes and compare information from the lecture with the textbook or handouts over the same topic. Schedule a 15-minute "preview" period to look over textual material on that topic just before lecture. Now aren't you glad you read the chapter on prereading while you were monitoring your time?

Be sure to schedule at least one hour of R&R every day. If, like many students starting a medical curriculum, you have discovered that you've been spending an inordinate amount of time in R&R and maintenance activities, it's tempting to swing too far the other direction and try to study "all the time." That is a mistake. Everyone needs to take time for some fun—every day if possible. "Fun" can be a walk or playing the piano or a bit of leisure reading. Just taking time to watch the sunset can be a real "upper" and give you the energy you need to get back to work with a will.

Also schedule at least two hours of heavy-duty physical exercise every week. (Ideally, we recommend a half-hour to an hour of physical activity every day.) Studying is too sedentary to be healthy without a program of planned exercise. Many students find that late afternoon is an excellent time for physical exercise. After a day of sitting and studying, most students feel an urge to move their muscles. Combined with the maintenance activity of preparing and eating dinner, late-afternoon exercise and dinner make an excellent break before settling into a period of concentrated study in the evening.

Plan at least one, and preferably two, periods of concentrated study on at least six days every week. Most students end up with a minimum of one longish (three hours) study period, plus one shorter period seven days a week during academic terms.

Continually recording how you use your time is the fastest and best way to improve your time management, according to experts on behavior management who deal with changing and controlling habits. How you use your time is a matter of habit and can be changed like any other habit. Until your desired schedule comes "naturally" (is a firm habit), keep recording your weekly totals. This will give you objective data about how your time is being spent.

Just as nobody is perfect, no plan is perfect. Be realistic in planning your schedule. If something important causes you to break from your plan, reschedule the original planned activity into another time slot that same week. The time rescheduled should be in the same category as the unplanned activity that preempted your original schedule. For instance, if you're invited on a great date for a time you originally scheduled as personal study time, you don't have to say, "I'm sorry, but your offer interferes with my plans to study histology that evening." You can accept with a clear conscience, if (and only if) you reschedule the same amount of personal study time into an R&R spot some other place on your weekly schedule. Try to keep your time swapping within the same week. Your schedule each week is too tight to borrow time from one week with the idea of repaying it the next. If you find yourself having to do a lot of schedule changing, either your schedule has not been well planned or you are impulsively jumping into unscheduled activities. The bottom line is this: The planned total hours for each activity should balance out by the end of the week, in the same way that (ideally) you balance your checkbook each month.

Don't clutter your weekly schedule with picky details. Put small details onto lists or into files. Grocery and errand lists are usually cleaned up weekly. About once a month, schedule two or three hours to take care of the items in your files.

Plan to get between 6 and 8 hours of sleep each night, including nights before exams. If you're regularly sleeping more than 8 hours in 24, you might want to remember that excessive sleep is sometimes a way of not dealing with issues such as stress or depression. It can also be a symptom of physical disease. If you tend to "borrow" sleep time or regularly deprive yourself of more than you need you will have to repay it with "interest" in the form of lost concentration, ill health, or both.

If you are married or have a special partner to share your life, plan to spend at least one evening each week plus a half-day each weekend with that person. Consider the time as high a priority as studying (with the possible exception of major examination periods, such as finals). It counts as R&R on your weekly schedule but counts as top value in life planning.

☞ **You are now ready to** *plan* **a good weekly schedule.**

Exercise 2: Planning a Weekly Schedule (Plan/Actual)

Tear out the perforated Plan/Actual Time-Monitoring Schedule (Table 1.4) and make as many copies as you need before you write on it. Now schedule in the "Plan" column all your high-priority activities, such as labs and lecture or small-group meetings. Also schedule other necessary activities: physical exercise, meals, sleep, and R&R. Mark on the Plan side when you want to do your personal study. Carry this schedule with you every day. You will need to

Table 1.4 Plan/Actual Time-Monitoring Schedule

Record your activities in one hour or in half-hour units for one week. At the end of the week, calculate totals for major activities using the following categories: LEC (lecture), LAB (laboratory), SLA (scheduled learning activities—e.g., seminars, review sessions), PS (personal study), JOB (employed hours), M (maintenance activities—shopping, cooking, cleaning, errands, eating, personal hygiene, etc.), PE (physical exercise), S (sleep), R&R (rest and recreation—anything that does not fit into previous categories).

Name _____

Week of _____

	Monday		Tuesday		Wednesday		Thursday		Friday		Saturday		Sunday	
	Plan	Actual	Plan	Actual	Plan	Actual	Plan	Actual	Plan	Actual	Plan	Actual	Plan	Actual
5:30 a.m.														
6:00														
6:30														
7:00														
7:30														
8:00														
9:00														
10:00														
11:00														
12:00 p.m.														
12:30														
1:00														
2:00														
3:00														
4:00														
5:00														

29

5:30								
6:00								
6:30								
7:00								
7:30								
8:00								
8:30								
9:00								
9:30								
10:00								
10:30								
11:00								
11:30								
12:00								
12:30								
1:00								
1:30								

Daily totals

All study					
Main					
PE					
R&R					
Sleep					

Weekly actual totals: Study = ___ ; Main = ___ ; PE = ___ ; R&R = ___ ; Sleep = ___

refer to it periodically to be sure you are following your plan. You'll feel positively noble as you check off completion of your plan each hour in the "Actual" column. If you did not follow your plan, make a note in the Actual column of what you really did with that unit of time. See the samples in Tables 1.5 and 1.6 for how two students recorded their planned and actual activities for one week.

While you are doing this second week of time monitoring, you may go on to Chapter 3, "Reading and Note Making." Again, we urge that you not go past this one chapter during the week.

At the end of the plan/actual time-monitoring week, return to this chapter and complete "Check-Up for Exercise 2: Plan/Actual Time Monitoring."

☞ You may go on to Chapter 3, "Reading and Note Making."

Check-Up for Exercise 2: Plan/Actual Time Monitoring

Briefly write your answers to the following questions, based on what you have learned from monitoring your time for the past week using the Plan/Actual Time-Monitoring Schedule.

1. How close did you come to your plan?

    _____

    _____

2. If you weren't close, why? What did you substitute for planned activities? Can you detect a pattern?

    _____

    _____

3. What further changes are necessary?

    _____

    _____

If you kept reasonably close to your planned schedule—**Congratulations!** You can now switch to a regular appointment book for scheduling activities.

(text continues on page 36)

Table 1.5 Linda R.'s Plan/Actual Time-Monitoring Schedule

Record your activities in one hour or in half-hour units for one week. At the end of the week, calculate totals for major activities using the following categories: LEC (lecture), LAB (laboratory), SLA (scheduled learning activities—e.g., seminars, review sessions), PS (personal study), JOB (employed hours), M (maintenance activities—shopping, cooking, cleaning, errands, eating, personal hygiene, etc.), PE (physical exercise), S (sleep), R&R (rest and recreation—anything that does not fit into previous categories).

Name _____ Linda R. _____

Week of _____ October 26–November 2 _____

	Monday		Tuesday		Wednesday		Thursday		Friday		Saturday		Sunday	
	Plan	Actual	Plan	Actual	Plan	Actual	Plan	Actual	Plan	Actual	Plan	Actual	Plan	Actual
5:30 a.m.	S		S		S		S		S		S		S	
6:00	M		M		M		M		M		S		S	
6:30	M		M		M		M		M		S		S	
7:00	M		M		M		M		M		M		S	
7:30	M		M		M		M		M		M		M	
8:00	LEC		LEC		PS		LEC		LEC		PS		M	
9:00	LEC		LEC		LEC		LEC		LEC		PS		M	
10:00	LAB		LAB		PS		LAB		PS		PS		M	
11:00	LAB		LAB		LEC		LAB		PS		PS		M	
12:00 p.m.	M		M		M		M		M		M		M	
12:30	PS	M	PS	R&R	PS	R&R	PS		PS	M	M		PS	PE
1:00	LEC		LEC		LEC		LEC		LEC		M		PS	
2:00	LAB		PS	R&R	LAB		LEC		LAB		PS		PS	
3:00	LAB		PS		LAB		PS		LAB		PS		PS	
4:00	PS		SLA		LAB		PS		LAB		PS		PS	

32

Weekly schedule grid (time slots 5:00 p.m. – 1:00 a.m.), with daily and weekly totals.

Time													
5:00	M			M	M	M		LAB		PS		PS	M
5:30	M			M	M	M	M	M	M	M	M	M	M
6:00	M			M	M	M	M	M	M	M	M	M	M
6:30	M			M	M	M	M	M	M	M	M	M	M
7:00	PS			PS	M	M	PS	M	PS	M	R&R	M	M
7:30	PS			PS	PS	M	PS	PS	R&R	R&R	R&R	R&R	M
8:00	PS			PS	PS	M	PS	PS	R&R	R&R	R&R	R&R	M
8:30	PS	M		PS	PS	M	PS	PS	PS		M	PS	M
9:00	PS			PS	PS	PS	PS	PS	PS	PS	PS	PS	M
9:30	PS			PS	PS	PS	PS	PS	PS	PS	PS	PS	M
10:00	PE			R&R	R&R	PS	PE	PE	R&R	R&R	PE	R&R	R&R
10:30	PS	M		R&R	R&R	M	PS	M	R&R		PS	R&R	R&R
11:00	M	M		M	M	S	M	S	M	S	M	M	M
11:30	S	S		S	S		S		S		M	M	S
12:00												S	
12:30													
1:00													

Daily totals

All study	12	10.5	12	11	11.5	10.5	10.5	10	12	10.5	9	8	6.5	4.5
Main	5	6.5	5	5	5	5.5	7	7	5	5.5	5	6	9	9
PE	.5	.5	.5	.5	0	0	0	.5	0	.5	.5	.5	0	1
R&R	0	0	0	1	1	1.5	0	0	0	1	2	2.5	1	2
Sleep	6.5	6.5	6.5	6.5	6.5	6.5	6.5	6.5	8	8	7.5	7.5	6.5	6.5

Weekly actual totals: Study = <u>65</u>; Main = <u>44</u>; PE = <u>3.5</u>; R&R = <u>8</u>; Sleep = <u>48</u>

Table 1.6 Kenneth B.'s Plan/Actual Time-Monitoring Schedule

Record your activities in one hour or in half-hour units for one week. At the end of the week, calculate totals for major activities using the following categories: LEC (lecture), LAB (laboratory), SLA (scheduled learning activities—e.g., seminars, review sessions), PS (personal study), JOB (employed hours), M (maintenance activities—shopping, cooking, cleaning, errands, eating, personal hygiene, etc.), PE (physical exercise), S (sleep), R&R (rest and recreation—anything that does not fit into previous categories).

Name: _____ Kenneth B. _____   Week of _____ January 24-30 _____

	Monday		Tuesday		Wednesday		Thursday		Friday		Saturday		Sunday	
	Plan	Actual	Plan	Actual	Plan	Actual	Plan	Actual	Plan	Actual	Plan	Actual	Plan	Actual
5:30 a.m.	S		S		S		S		S		S		S	
6:00	S		S		S		S		S		S		S	
6:30	S		S		M	S	S		M	S	M	S	S	
7:00	M		M		M	S	M		M		M	PE	M	
7:30	M		M		PS	M	M		M		PS	M	M	
8:00	LEC		LEC		PS	M	LEC		LEC		PS	M	M	R&R
9:00	LEC		LEC		LEC		LEC		LEC		PS		R&R	
10:00	LAB		LEC		LEC		LAB		LAB		PS		R&R	
11:00	LAB		PS		LEC		LAB		LAB		PS		R&R	
12:00 p.m.	M		M		M		M		M		M		M	
12:30	PS	M	PS		PS		PS	M	PS	M	PS	M	PE	
1:00	LAB		PS		PS		PS		PS		PS		PE	
2:00	LAB		LAB		PS		LAB		PS		PS		PE	
3:00	LAB		LAB		PS		LAB		PS		PS	PE	PE	R&R
4:00	LAB		PS	M	SLA		PS		PS	M	PS		R&R	

Daily totals

All study	12.5	12	13.5	9.5	12	9.5	12	11.5	10.5	9	5.5	0	0
Main	2	3	3	5.5	2	4.5	3.5	2.5	3	.5	5	4	4
PE	1.5	1	1	1	1	1	1	1	1.5	1.5	5	2	2
R&R	.5	.5	0	1.5	1.5	1.5	0	1	2	6	6.5	9.5	10.5
Sleep	7.5	7.5	6.5	6.5	7.5	7.5	7.5	8	7.5	7	6.5	7.5	8

Weekly actual totals: Study = <u>58</u>; Main = <u>28.5</u>; PE = <u>8</u>; R&R = <u>22.5</u>; Sleep = <u>51.5</u>

Buy one that fits easily into your backpack, briefcase, purse, or whatever you carry around with you all day.

If your actual time spent was *not* close to what you had planned, you could benefit from another week of completing the Plan/Actual Time-Monitoring Schedule. Revise your plan for the next week, using this experience and analysis, and do a second week of plan/actual time monitoring.

It's interesting to think about how to accomplish your goals with maximum efficiency. You may have developed some slick tricks of your own to save time. Here are some time-saving tips gleaned from busy students who manage to remember friends and family, do all the "dumb things you have to do," keep clean and fed, and still spend 60 to 65 hours each week in learning activities.

Time-Savers

1. Do two things at the same time, but only if neither requires special concentration:
   - Listen to the news while preparing meals, doing your hair, shaving, or ironing clothes. Exercise while watching your favorite TV program.
   - Sort through note cards (see chapter on note making) while waiting for something/someone.
   - Combine exercise with socializing. Walk, jog, or go to the gym with a friend.
   - Combine necessary nonacademic activities with socializing (sharing a meal with a friend is a classic example).
2. Go low maintenance:
   - Buy low-maintenance clothing.
   - Get a "wash and wear" hairstyle.
   - Select food that requires little preparation. Eating "raw" or "plain" food is usually healthier, too.
3. Keep lists for all regular/routine maintenance activities:
   - Put items on a list as soon as you know you will be out within a week to avoid extra trips to the store.
   - Maintain a weekly errand list and combine as many trips as are practical. Schedule errands on an efficient route to minimize time and mileage.
4. Always carry your daily schedule book with you:
   - Attach a Post-it™ note pad to the inside cover to make temporary notes as needed.
   - Clip a pen or pencil inside the cover.

5. Keep a "pending" file and sort through it once a month. Put in any item you think you might want to keep but aren't quite sure about using later. If you haven't referred to it or used it after a month or two, toss it in the trash. This is the one case where procrastination can pay! And it keeps your desk space uncluttered.

6. Keep an "unanswered letters" file. Schedule a regular time to write letters. When you're busy, answer in very brief notes. Buy small-sized stationery, note cards, or postcards for this purpose. You can use Post-it notes for ideas to put in your replies as they occur to you and save your gems until you're ready to send your next note. Or telephone, if you can afford it (both time and money). E-mail can be a real time-saver if you have Internet access. Do be aware of the passage of time, though. Set a timer to keep yourself on schedule if this is a problem for you.

7. Keep an "unpaid bills" file for depositing all those statements that come in the mail. Go through this file every two weeks. Bills unpaid past the deadline often cost you extra time, money, and headaches—another desktop cleaner-upper. Or to cut down on the number of bills you have to physically deal with each month, consider automatic payments from your bank or credit union checking account.

8. Keep a current, alphabetical list of all people and businesses important in your life. Most commercial schedule books have a place for names, addresses, and telephone numbers. Use your annual schedule book to keep track of birthdays, anniversaries, or other dates you need to remember. Move them forward at the end of the year to next year's schedule book. You'll save last-minute trips for gifts and cards by getting them worked into your weekly errand list. If you use an electronic calendar, you can have it remind you in advance of when to buy and mail the card, too!

9. Keep a "health" file with all dental, medical, and optometry records so that you can find them quickly when needed.

10. Have a regular, assigned place for everything. This applies especially to small articles that you constantly pick up and put down again: keys, glasses, watches, wallets, pens.

11. Do things when other people don't. This applies to movies (go at 5 p.m. and eat afterward), grocery shopping (avoid 6 p.m.), driving during peak commuter hours.

12. Think if you drink. Stop before the next day is "blown" while you recover from the physiological damage of too much alcohol.

13. Protect your personal study time. When friends interrupt your study in public places—for example, at the library—tell them you'd really enjoy having a good visit, and then pull out your schedule book and write in a

date to get together. Or you can say you plan to take a 10-minute break at a specific time and would enjoy a chat during that break. When the telephone interrupts your concentrated study period at home, you have several options:

- Don't answer if you have an answering machine. You can call back later when it's convenient. If you don't have one, put an answering machine on your birthday list!
- If you know you can discipline yourself to answer very briefly, answer and close the call within a minute or two.
- If you can't stand not answering the phone when it rings, turn off the ringer or unplug it during study periods.

14. Question spending time in study groups among friends. Much of the time is spent socializing rather than studying. Use the 50-minute rule to decide if the group is really studying. If more than 10 minutes of an hour in the study group is spent off the topic, then you'd have to count it as R&R, not study time.

Exercise 3: What Have You Learned?

What was the main thing you learned from working your way through this chapter on time management?

Students Say

"The time questionnaires made me realize how I waste my time."

"It's now clear to me that I need to spend more time working with the material."

"My time is limited, and I have to make the best use of each block due to personal commitments—no leeway." (This from a new mother.)

"I needed the time management skills (and time-monitoring sheets) the first week of medical school!" (This from a student in second term of medical school.)

"I need to have a schedule of what I am to do with myself at all times and follow it."

"I found out I was wasting my 'in-between' time and was sleeping too much as a stress-reliever."

"I felt more responsible and more aware of my time. My time had been slipping away."

"I've been spending far too much time on nonessential things. I got better about this at the end. I was spending too much time on maintenance activities."

"I learned I need to use my R&R time to better advantage—for example, to exercise, rather than just waste time."

"Keeping a schedule forces me to manage my time better."

"It's easy to let an hour slip by and it becomes R&R instead of study time. I thought I was studying a lot more than I really was."

Outcomes

Of the hundreds of students who have participated in our workshops, we have been able to collect data over a period of several years about use of time before the workshop and again at the end from medical and veterinary medical students at three different schools. In the aggregate, they averaged 41.8 total hours of study per week, including lectures, labs, and personal study, during the baseline period, which we used as a pretest. At the end of the workshop, the students averaged 60.5 hours per week in learning activities. Further analysis revealed two quite different groups of students. One group did not allocate enough time at the beginning of the program. Indeed, some were surprised when their baseline showed only 6 to 10 hours of personal study time per week, using the 50-minute rule. This group needed to devote more time to personal study. The other group actually improved their study habits by decreasing the amount of time spent in personal study. They were inefficient and wasted time staring at textbooks and notes or not really paying attention at lectures. Using information in the chapters on previewing, concentration, and note making, they learned more in less time!

Summary

Most medical students must make a major adjustment in their use of time as they begin medical school. To have enough time to cover and review the mass of information presented in medical classes, students need to spend, on the average, between 60 and 65 hours every week in learning activities. Much depends on the quality of premedical preparation. Not all students enter medical school with the same background. Obviously, someone with an undergraduate biochemistry major will not have to spend the same amount of time on the basic medical biochemistry course as the student who has never encountered it before. Students with weaker premedical preparation may need to schedule more than 65 hours a week to get a good start in medical school but can build a foundation from this extra study that will permit them to catch up with their classmates in the first two years.

The exercises in this chapter provided an opportunity for you to determine how you have been spending your time. Suggestions were offered for more effective time management, and you were encouraged to customize this advice to meet your own specific needs. Planning and following a schedule can have the additional benefit of helping to free you from much of the stress that seems to be part of the hectic life of medical students.

If You Want to Know More

Colvin, R. H., & Taylor, D. D. (1978). Planning student work-study time in an objectives-based medical curriculum. *Journal of Medical Education, 53,* 393-396.

   Authors advocate a formula for calculating time necessary for learning activities.

Crissey, G. (1987). Responses to survey of time spent in academic activities. Internal report, College of Veterinary Medicine, Cornell University, Ithaca, New York.

   From a survey conducted by the college registrar, first-year veterinary medical students spent an average of 26.1 hours in class and laboratory per week and an average of 33.7 hours per week in personal study, totaling 59.8 hours in learning activities each week. Second-year students were scheduled for 26.9 hours of lecture and laboratory and reported spending 41.7 hours in personal study weekly—a total of 68.6 hours in all learning activities.

Davis, W. K., & Heller, L. E. (1976). The effects of a demanding curriculum on students' allocation of time. *Journal of Medical Education, 51,* 506-507.

A 28-day study of 19 sophomore medical students at the University of Michigan Medical School. There was a strong positive correlation between amount of study time and grades. Average total time in personal study and classes was 60 hours.

Fisher, L. A., & Cotsonas, N. J. A. (1965). Time study of student activities. *Journal of Medical Education, 40,* 125-131.

Time monitored in "educational activities" totaled 65 hours per week—25 hours per week in class and 41 hours per week in other study activities.

Garrard, J., Lorents, A., & Chilgren, R. (1972). Student allocation of time in a semioptional medical curriculum. *Journal of Medical Education, 47,* 460-466.

A 21-day study of random observations of 21 medical students. Students scheduled 31.8 hours per week by the school for organized learning activities. Students recorded a total of 110.96 hours in all activities, including personal time, transit, personal study, and patient-related work.

Jesse, W. F., & Simon, H. J. (1971). Time utilization by medical students on a pass/fail evaluation system. *Journal of Medical Education, 46,* 275-280.

Average time in educational activities totaled 62 hours per week. Students tended to overestimate time requirements of the program and to underestimate leisure time.

Kelman, E. (1978). Stressors for veterinary medical students and types of students reporting most stress. *Journal of Veterinary Medical Education, 5*(3), 145-151.

Time pressure was a major stress for veterinary medical students who typically spend 60 hours per week in study activities.

2 Prereading as a Way to Maximize Usefulness of Lecture Time

(Week 1)

Student: When I go to lecture I don't understand half the words the professor is using! How can I even take notes?

Mentor: Have you tried prereading?

Student: There is no way I could read the whole assignment before I go to lecture. I'm lucky just to get there on time.

Mentor: That's not prereading. Let me explain. . . .

Before reading Chapter 2, take a few minutes for a diagnosis:

Diagnose Yourself: Prereading Before a Lecture

Directions: Circle the number that best describes your actual behavior during an academic term.

Never
Rarely
Sometimes
Often
Always

0 1 2 3 4   1. I prepare in advance for lectures by prereading textual materials on the upcoming lecture topic.

0 1 2 3 4   2. Before a lecture, I have identified the main ideas related to the lecture topic.

0 1 2 3 4   3. Before a lecture, I know the name and spelling of key details of the lecture topic.

43

01 2 3 4   4. Before a lecture, I have some idea of the relationship between main ideas and their key details; for example, I would know in advance if the topic involves a time sequence, cause and effect, or contrasting and comparing subtopics.

01 2 3 4   5. My previewing of textual material prior to a lecture is accomplished rapidly (at a rate of 10-15 minutes per hour of lecture).

0 1 2 3 4   6. Before a lecture, I have a general idea of the format my condensed notes will take (diagrams, flowcharts, category charts, cards, outlines, or some combination of the above).

4 3 2 1 0   7. I fall asleep during lecture.

4 3 2 1 0   8. After a lecture, I spend too much time making a set of condensed notes for review.

4 3 2 1 0   9. I find it hard to follow what the lecturer is saying.

4 3 2 1 0   10. I find it hard to concentrate during a lecture.

4 3 2 1 0   11. The vocabulary in a lecture is new to me.

0 1 2 3 4   12. I spend 10 to 15 minutes looking over what will be covered in a lecture that day or the next day.

25   **Total score** (sum of circled items)

☞ Stop.
Do not continue until you are
ready to score the prereading assessment.

Scoring Directions: Prereading Diagnosis

Directions: Add all the numbers you circled for the total score.

1. If you prepare in advance for lectures by prereading the upcoming lecture topic, you will be able to better organize the material during the lecture. This will save time later during your personal study period. You can also better understand a less than perfectly organized lecture.

2. Identifying the main ideas related to the lecture topic enables you to better organize the material.

3. Knowing the name and spelling of key words of the lecture topic facilitates note taking during lecture.

4. If you have some idea of the relationship between main ideas and their key details in advance (if the topic involves a time sequence, cause and effect, or contrasting and comparing subtopics along similar dimensions), your comprehension and retention of the material is enhanced. You also have a head start on creating your own set of organized notes for later review.

5. Spending longer than 10 to 15 minutes in prereading, is not prereading—it is *reading!* Spending less than 10 minutes may not give an adequate overview.

6. If before lecture you have a general idea of the format your condensed notes will take (diagrams, flowcharts, category charts, cards, outlines, or some combination), you speed up the process of making those notes.

7. Falling asleep during a lecture may be due to inactivity (if not lack of sleep). Becoming more **active** in your learning and note taking will help keep you awake. Also, people are usually more interested in a topic they already have studied—even if the study is only the preview given by 10 minutes of prereading.

8. About 50% to 60% of your personal study time will probably be spent in making your set of condensed notes for review. Spending longer than this will cut into your review and self-test time, which is the key to a good study system.

9. Following what a lecturer says is easier if you have an idea of where he or she is going, based on your prereading of the topic. You can impose organization even on an unorganized lecture.

10. Concentration during a lecture is improved by anticipating what will come next and being actively engaged in note making.

11. The vocabulary in a lecture will not be new to you if you preread the material.

12. Spending 10 to 15 minutes prereading what will be covered in a lecture will give you a head start on making your condensed review note *during a lecture.*

Score Interpretation: Prereading Diagnosis

If your score was 36 or above, you're doing fine. **Congratulations!** If your score was 35 or below, prereading can help you learn more during the hours of lecture you hear every week.

Making the Most of Lecture Time

Lectures are medieval—that is, a way of learning before printed books were available to students. You can probably "cover" the same material more rapidly by reading or by using computer-assisted instructional software. But most students *do* choose to attend lecture in medical school for these reasons:

- Lecturers highlight **what will be on the test** (almost always), and that is certainly what most students fervently desire to know. Lecturers cover what they think is important (and what they think is important is more likely to **be on the test**) or give you their angle on the main topics, which are likely to **be on the test.**

- Lecturers occasionally add to information given in the syllabus or text— examples or new, "up-to-the-minute" information. If they go to the trouble of adding something extra, odds are high that it will also **be on the test.**

Close to 70% of what you must learn about any topic will typically be presented in the lectures. Prereading will help you save time because you'll actually learn more during all those hours of sitting in lectures. Because many students spend about 20 hours a week in lecture, the question arises, "How well is this time being used?" Are you (a) asleep, (b) half-asleep, or (c) alert and taking notes but playing stenographer without knowing shorthand, missing half of the lecture because you're writing so much?

Many students waste a good portion of lecture time—not concentrating, not getting good notes, not really learning, or not preparing to learn while in lecture. It's inefficient not to get at least a tentative version of good, condensed, self-testable notes while attending lecture so that personal study time can be devoted more to review and self-test. And you'd need less personal study time if the many hours of lecture time were optimally used.

The key to really learning in lecture and leaving the lecture hall with a usable set of notes is **prereading.** Another benefit: Studies show that prereading increases later reading rate (when you return to the text after the lecture) an average of 25% at the same time that comprehension of the topic increases by 10%. That's efficient!

What Is Prereading?

- **Rapid skimming.** It should not take more than 10 to 15 minutes to preread for an hour's worth of lecture material; if it does, you're not prereading—you're *reading!*
- **Looking for the "big picture"** or main points in the text. Is there a unifying concept?

- **Getting a sense of the vocabulary,** learning new terms that will appear in the lecture and in later focused reading.
- **Spotting the patterns** of relationships between subtopics and main topics.
- **Analyzing** causes and effects, comparisons and contrasts, the time sequencing, and so on.

How to Preread

You may preread from a variety of materials:

- Textbook
- Course syllabus
- Old class notes (previous year)
- Review books

Obviously you can't preread from every source available. It's important to find the best one or two sources for each class.

If a note service is available (and course content is the same or similar to the previous year), you may choose to preread last year's notes and take them with you to lecture. You need write only new notes about additional information or changes from the previous year. This will reduce the amount of writing, yet keep you actively involved in the lecture.

When you preread, notice the following:

- Study questions—read these first then scan for the answers
- First paragraph
- Bold-faced print
- Subtitles
- Colored print
- Italicized print
- Shaded areas
- Boxed information
- Diagrams
- Charts
- Tables

- Graphs
- Lists
- Pictures
- Glossary of new terms
- Summary
- Objectives
- First sentence of paragraphs

Prereading encourages active (vs. passive) learning to take place—anticipating what is coming instead of just letting it "wash over you" and hoping that some will stick.

While prereading look for the following:

- Key ideas
- Main subordinate details
- Relationships between key ideas and details
- Relationships between key ideas (enumeration, comparison, contrast, time sequence, cause and effect, classification)

When is the best time of day or week to preread? Usually in the evening prior to the next morning's lectures. Some students prefer to preread immediately before a lecture, but because most lectures are scheduled in the morning, that would necessitate being an extra-early riser.

Exercise 1: Prereading— Making the Best Use of Lecture Time

Directions: Select a chapter from any text that will be covered in lecture within the next couple of days (preferably tomorrow). You will preview this chapter in 10 minutes.

Before you begin, read these guidelines for prereading:

- Keep your book flat on the table in front of you.
- Put both hands on your book or other reading material. Have one hand ready to turn the page.

- Preview the section to be read. See if you can glean the general outline in two or three minutes. Then go back and look at titles, subheadings, summary, and review questions. Previewing the section tells you what to look for as you preread. Give yourself a purpose for your reading and a reason to remember what you've read.
- Don't take notes.
- Don't pause much for numbers or tables.
- Look for the basic concepts, not the details.
- Look for cues that indicate most important ideas and terms (headlines, indentations, outlines, italics, bold, underlining).
- Don't reread anything. Don't go back over material you've already covered.
- Move your eyes down the page as fast as you can. Your goal is to move through these pages as quickly as possible. You should feel a slight tension about getting through this material in the time you've allowed.

Check your watch or clock and give yourself no more than 10 minutes to preread the section you've chosen. Count the number of pages before you begin, so you'll know how to pace yourself. Return to Check-Up for Exercise 1 when you've finished.

☞ Start prereading now.
Stop after 10 minutes
Go to Check-Up for Exercise 1

Check-Up for Exercise 1: Prereading—Making the Best Use of
Lecture Time

1. List the main point(s) in the chapter or section you selected.

   prefixes, suffixes, eponyms, combining forms, abbreviations.

2. If there's more than one main point, what is the relationship between them?

   how they can be used together to create medical terminology.

3. List some of the key details.

Vowels can be used to combine prefixes &
suffixes, words can be derived from names
of those who discovered them.

4. How are these details related to a key point?

Related b/c explaining how words are
made or derived

Although few medical students read textual material before a lecture, several research studies show that prereading increases comprehension and puts information into longer-term memory. Students are also able to identify what is important and on exams are able to give better answers to higher-order questions.

Prereading is like looking at the road map before going on a trip. You will know ahead of time where the route changes and place names along the way. As looking at a map before a trip is an advance organizer for your journey, prereading is an advance organizer for the topic you are about to study. It's all right that you don't have detailed knowledge from prereading. You'll cover it again in lecture. And you'll return for more focused reading after the lecture when you create your set of condensed notes for review.

Exercise 2: Prereading for One Week

Prove to yourself how useful prereading can be! Preread for your lecture classes next week. Lectures are usually scheduled in the morning with only a few minutes break between them, so the best time to preread for morning lectures is probably the night before. You can preread for afternoon lectures during a midday break. The point is to have the ideas fresh in your mind as you listen to the lecture.

☞ **During this week of prereading,
start the next chapter,
"Reading and Note Making."
Then return to this chapter
for the Check-Up on Exercise 2.**

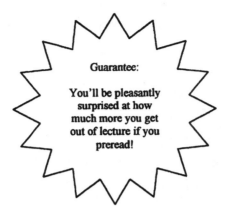

Guarantee:

You'll be pleasantly surprised at how much more you get out of lecture if you preread!

Check-Up for Exercise 2: Prereading for One Week

1. List what prereading accomplished in terms of gain from lecture time.

_____

_____

2. List other benefits of prereading.

_____

_____

After prereading for a week, we hope you'll be as enthusiastic as other students who have become converts to this study strategy.

Students Say

"I knew what the lecturer was talking about!"

"I knew where he was going with the topic."

"I could spell the words she used."

"I could organize the material even when it wasn't presented in an organized way."

"I stayed awake."

"It makes all the difference!"

"Makes class interesting."

"Makes you feel intelligent!"

Summary

Prereading is the first of the four steps in the *Study Without Stress* system. It has three main benefits. Students who preread

- comprehend more from their many hours of lecture time,
- have longer retention rate of information,
- get a jump start on creating their own set of study notes, which is the topic of the next chapter.

If You Want to Know More

Cook, L. K., & Mayer, R. E. (1988). Teaching readers about the structure of a scientific text. *Journal of Educational Psychology, 80,* 448-456.

College biology students showed substantial gains in recall of high conceptual information when they had previously noted the organization of information presented in the text: enumeration, sequence, or comparison and contrast.

Jacobowitz, T. (1981). The effects of modified skimming on college students' recall and recognition of expository text. In *Directions in reading: Research and instruction* (pp. 232-237). Washington, DC: National Reading Conference.

Advance knowledge of the text facilitates understanding. Skimming provides insight into the text by exposing the reader to many of the major points intended by the author.

Karlin, R. (1969). *Reading for achievement* (see pp. 3-25). New York: Holt, Rinehart & Winston.

Provides detailed instructions on how to preread.

Krug, D., George, B., Hannon, S. A., & Glover, J. A. (1989). The effect of outlines and headings on readers' recall of text. *Contemporary Educational Psychology, 14*(2), 111-123.

Students who read outlines prior to reading the texts recall information better on later tests.

Quirk, M. E. (1994). *How to learn and teach in medical school.* Springfield, IL: Charles C Thomas.

Strongly recommends previewing for meaning prior to reading and gives instructions on previewing skills.

Redding, R. E. (1990). Metacognitive instruction: Trainers teaching thinking skills. *Performance Improvement Quarterly, 3*(1), 27-41.

Critical review of research in metacognition and recommendations for assessing and facilitating metacognitive skills.

Snapp, J. C., & Glover, J. A. (1990). Advance organizers and study questions. *Journal of Educational Research, 83*(51), 266-271.

Students who read and paraphrased advance organizers gave significantly better answers to higher-order study questions.

Spencer, F., Johnston, M., & Ames, W. (1981). The effect of manipulating the advance organizer and other prereading strategies on comprehension of abstract text. In *Directions in reading: Research and instruction* (pp. 228-231). Washington, DC: National Reading Conference.

An overview can significantly increase the processing of unfamiliar or abstract material, especially if the material is not well organized.

Tudor, Ian. (1986). Advance organisers as adjuncts to reading comprehension. *Journal of Research in Reading, 9*(2), 103-115.

Experiment showed advance organizers—that is, a prior overview of textual information—facilitates comprehension especially for more complex texts. The greater the level of textual difficulty, the more benefit advance organizers provide.

Wade, S. E., & Reynolds, R. E. (1989). Developing metacognitive awareness. *Journal of Reading, 33*(1), 6-14.

> *Deciding what to study, or "what is important," is a key component to skillful reading. Skilled learners pay extra attention to main ideas of the text and are aware of textual clues that point to key ideas. The clues are headings, topic sentences, amount of space author gives to the idea, bold-faced print, italicized print, lists, and study questions provided.*

3 Reading and Note Making

(Week 2)

Student: I spend all of my time studying but still have trouble on the tests. What am I doing wrong?

Mentor: What do you do when you study?

Student: I read the material and highlight what I think is important with a pink highlighter. Then I go back through and mark with blue highlighter what seems most important of the already highlighted part. So when I review for tests I concentrate on the purple portions, those highlighted first in pink and later in blue. Here, let me show you. (Digs through backpack and pulls out physiology text.)

Mentor (flipping through the pink, blue, and purple textbook): Very colorful!

Highlighting as you read *is* better than just reading. But most students don't have time to review all the material they've highlighted, because they've highlighted half the text. In this chapter, you will learn how to make a condensed, organized set of notes that is easy to review and use for self-testing before examinations. Usually, this chapter is completed during the second week of time monitoring.

Before reading this chapter, take a few minutes to *diagnose yourself.*

Diagnose Yourself: Reading and Note Making

Directions: Circle the number that best describes your actual behavior during an academic term.

Never
Rarely
Sometimes
Often
Always

4 (3) 2 1 0   1. I highlight and/or underline as much as a third of each page of my textbooks.

0 1 (2) 3 4   2. I rewrite/organize my notes immediately (within one or two days) following the lecture.

(4) 3 2 1 0   3. I don't understand some parts of what I am studying.

0 1 2 3 (4)   4. I make notes on a separate sheet of paper or in a notebook as I read my textbooks.

0 1 2 3 (4)   5. I condense my notes into outlines, tables, charts, diagrams, or cards to facilitate review.

0 1 2 3 (4)   6. I organize my condensed notes so that supporting details are placed into the context of main ideas covered in the lecture or text.

0 1 2 3 (4)   7. I write condensed notes in a format that I can review easily and quickly.

0 1 2 3 (4)   8. I design condensed notes so that I can use them later to test myself over the information.

0 1 (2) 3 4   9. I use flash cards to memorize important details that my self-test reveals I do not recall easily.

4 (3) 2 1 0   10. I get lost in the details of the subject I'm studying and "can't see the forest for the trees."

4 (3) 2 1 0   11. I find it hard to distinguish the more important information from less important details.

0 1 2 3 (4)   12. I note relationships among themes or topics as I study.

0 1 2 3 (4)   13. I see how details fit into the "big picture" of the topic I'm studying.

0 1 2 (3) 4   14. I organize my notes so that relationships among details "jump up" at me as I review them.

(4) 3 2 1 0   15. When I am studying, I am not sure how to organize the material so that I will see and remember meaningful associations on the test.

52   **Total score** (sum of circled items)

☞ Stop.
Do not continue until you are ready
to score the note-making assessment.

Scoring Directions: Reading and Note-Making Diagnosis

Add up all your circled answers and then sum the column totals for a total score.

1. If you highlight and/or underline as much as a third of each page of your textbooks, there will be too much material to review. Also, highlighting does not lend itself to self-testing or identifying information you are not remembering. Finally, highlighting does not organize information into memorable contexts. The value of highlighting is to focus attention on important information, but this value is lost if too much of the text is highlighted.

2. If you rewrite and organize your notes within one or two days of the lecture, you will always be caught up and will not have to "cram" before an exam, and the information from the lecture and reading will still be fresh and vivid in your thoughts.

3. If you're thinking, "I don't understand," you probably need to go through the process of very organized note making to see the relationships among the information presented. See the section later in this chapter titled "What to Do When You Don't Understand Something You Are Studying." It has tips to help you figure out what to do when you don't understand the information well enough to make any notes.

4. Making notes on a separate sheet of paper or in a notebook as you read your textbooks allows you to "cut yourself free" of the text, to condense and organize the information in the best possible way for you to learn it, and to put the information into a format so that you can check whether you have, in fact, learned it.

5. If you condense your notes into outlines, tables, charts, diagrams, or cards, both review and self-testing are easy. Research on learning shows that metacognition (perceiving the nature of the information to be learned) and contextual organization are keys to understanding and recall.

6. Highly organized condensed notes facilitate the task of learning and memorizing, both because of the context of association and because the notes can be reviewed repeatedly, which embeds them in memory.

7. Writing condensed notes in a format that you can review easily and quickly will encourage you to review your notes more often. Repetition is the key to memory.

8. Making condensed notes that you can use later to test yourself over the information is an efficient way to "zero in" on the details you do not recall ✓ and to give them more emphasis in future review.

9. Flash cards are portable and easy to sort, allowing you to continually spend your time on what you *don't* know. Reviewing them often during ✓ the day will help you memorize important details that self-testing reveals you do not recall easily.

10. Organizing review notes so that important details fit into the main themes ✓ solves this problem. There is a *pattern* to the way different trees grow in a forest!

11. As you read material for your class, constantly ask yourself, "What kind of information is this?" See the section later in this chapter titled, "Types ✓ of Notes Useful for Review and Self-Testing" for what to do after you answer this very important question.

12. Noting relationships among themes or topics as you study means you are ✓ actively studying and organizing the material as you go along.

13. Keeping the overall picture in mind helps you organize and remember the ✓ significant details.

14. To review your notes repeatedly (and this is crucial to memory), it is necessary to review them quickly. Your organizational principle and use of color, boxes, or other visual aids allow you to get your eyes over your ✓ notes rapidly.

15. The decision-making process about how to organize the information so that you will see its significance and remember it on the test is a major part of learning how to learn. If you are constantly deciding how to organize the facts to enhance your understanding and memory of the ✓ material through meaningful associations, you will be able to make your notes quickly and, having good notes, you will be in a position to review and test yourself over the information.

Score Interpretation: Reading and Note-Making Diagnosis

53-60 = Very good
45-52 = Good but could use improvement
35-44 = Need help
Below 34 = Desperate need—*This chapter will be a lifesaver for you!*

Regardless of your score, do yourself a favor and read this chapter. You may think you make good notes now, but in our experience, even good note takers have what we call "loose" notes. These are not as well organized and not as easily used for review and self-testing as the methods recommended here. Even the best note makers are constantly looking for ways to improve.

Don't let this be your definition of note taking—the transfer of the professor's lecture to the student's notebook without passing through the student's brain.

What to Do When You Don't Understand Something You Are Studying

Before making your notes, you must have at least a basic understanding of the topic you are studying (although making a good set of notes sometimes adds depth to that understanding). If you are seriously clueless about a topic that is likely to be important, the following procedure has, to our knowledge, always been successful.

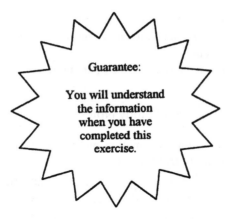

Guarantee:

You will understand the information when you have completed this exercise.

First, go to the medical library. Find the section of textbooks on the topic with which you are having difficulty. Select three to five standard textbooks likely to include an explanation (choose recent editions, standard references, texts that strike you as having an attractive format or layout). Using the index to find the right page(s), open each book to the page(s) covering that topic. You'll need a fair amount of space to lay out that many open books at once. Finally, read each explanation or discussion of the topic.

Each book explains the subject in a slightly different way and has a different set of illustrations and examples. Either the cumulative effect of reading multiple explanations or the particular approach of one of the authors should make this "click" for you so that you understand the information enough to begin your note making.

The Importance of Carefully Designed, Self-Testable, Condensed Notes

Here's why you need a set of carefully designed, self-testable notes:

- There is too much material to reread—even just what is highlighted.
- Without them, you can't get repeated, spaced review, which is the key to accurate and detailed recall.
- It's not possible to self-test from marginal notes or highlighted sections, so you can't assess what information needs more intense review.

Notes need to be in an easily reviewed and self-testable format to be useful. You really can't know that you know the material until you have tested yourself on the content.

OK, now that you're convinced, **let's get started.**

What Makes a Good Set of Study Notes?

- Clues to all essential information on the topic—the standard medical student problem of identifying what's important
- Highly organized information, in a format that reflects organically the logical relationships among the pieces of information to be remembered
- Visual interest so that ideas jump up from the page and are therefore more memorable
- Material condensed enough so that it is possible to review it repeatedly
- A format that permits self-testing because you can't be sure you know the material until you have successfully tested yourself on it

Notes should encourage an elaborated approach to information. This method avoids memorizing discrete bits just for the next exam and places knowledge into the more interesting context of conceptual wholes that will be continually useful in the future (e.g., finals, boards, clinical rotations). Research studies show that information organized into meaningful patterns is more easily remembered. Students seem to enjoy and have pride in working with the notes they have created.

After many years of observing students' notes for a variety of medical classes, we have identified several types. Each has its own special uses.

Types of Notes Useful for
Review and Self-Testing

Cards

Cards are one of the most common types of note making from premedical school years. They are still helpful in medical school. They're useful for multiple repetitions of specific details from your charts. They can also be used for remembering pieces of information that don't warrant a more complex form of note making. Examples are formulas, definitions, or enumerated information.

Cards should always be designed with a cue (or a question) on one side and the answer (or information to be remembered) on the other side (see Figures 3.1 and 3.2). Cards are the easiest kinds of notes for self-testing. They're portable, and they're simple in design.

Cards can be organized by grouping them under topics by rubber band or color coding by using different colored cards for different subjects. Self-testing is accomplished by going through a banded set and answering the questions. As you go through your cards, place those you easily answered correctly into a "know" pile. Place those you agonized over or just didn't know into a "don't know" pile. Thus, a topic is constantly sorted at each review, and each time, more cards will be added to the "know" pile until there is nothing left in the "don't know" pile. If you get into the habit of always carrying with you at least 10 cards from your "don't know" stack, you'll find many occasions every day to review them rapidly. Time that would otherwise be wasted (such as standing in line at the grocery or cafeteria, breaks between classes, waiting to meet a friend, etc.) can become time for one more repetition of detailed information. By the end of the day, you should be able to put all the cards you were carrying and reviewing into your "know" stack. At the end of a week, you'll have learned 60 to 70 new details at the rate of 10 cards a day. In a semester, that amounts to 900 to 1,000 bits of information learned during time that otherwise probably would have been wasted.

Store cards for future use. If you created them for a midterm, you will also have them to review for the final exam. They can be kept banded by topic or you can buy file boxes, use dividers, and label them for storage.

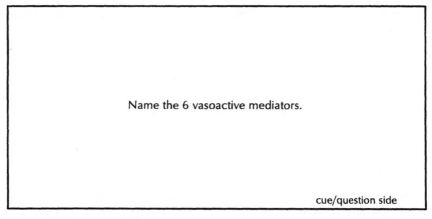

Figure 3.1. Front of card

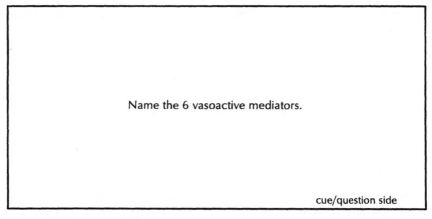

Figure 3.2. Back of card

Advantages and Disadvantages

The major advantages of cards are that (a) they are the best way to zero in on details you don't remember and (b) they're easy to sort. Although memorization is sometimes not much admired as an intellectual endeavor, there are a lot of details to be remembered in medical science, and cards are great for memorizing! The disadvantage of cards is that they lack the contextual cues to memory that are present in the more complex charts we'll describe next.

Category Charts

Category charts are excellent for information you want to compare and contrast. Usually there are three to seven similar types of details about each variable. For example, in pharmacology, you might want to compare and contrast the mechanism of action, indication, contraindication, and dose in a certain class of drugs. If they're clustered according to the mechanism of action, some general principles about the relationships within the class of drugs become apparent.

Unless otherwise noted, the sample charts reproduced here (see Figures 3.3, 3.4, and 3.5) are actual charts created by a student while he was enrolled in medical school. They represent the student's perception of "what's important to know" and are probably not perfect. Neither the creator of the charts nor the authors can take responsibility for the accuracy of the technical information contained in the charts used as examples in this book. These are simply examples of a student's attempts to organize material. We hope you will find them valuable even though they were not created by subject matter experts. Category charts created by experts, however, frequently appear in textbooks to summarize and organize information.

Anything that can be outlined can be charted according to categories. The main headings down the left column are usually equivalent to the roman numerals or capital letters of an outline. Across the top of the chart are the categories of information you want to remember, which usually correspond in outline form to the indented arabic numbers. In the cells or boxes that form the intersections of main headings and categories of information are written the details you want to remember. Category charts can be useful in practically any medical course you are taking.

Tips From Students on Making Category Charts

- Don't start the final chart until after attending lecture and reading the text on that topic.
- Make a tentative chart after previewing and during lecture. Consider using the course objectives from the syllabus or outline, headings, summary, and study questions in text to form headings for rows and columns.
- The organization of the lecture is a good clue to main concepts that should be column and row headings. Look for key words related to each concept.
- Sometimes a graph or table in the text provides a "ready-made" chart. Use it!

MECHANISM	PROTECTION	PATHOLOGY
HUMORAL		
Neutralization	• Toxins • Blocks Viral Receptors	• Insulin Resistance
Cytotoxic	• Bacteriolysis • ADCC • Opsonization	• RBC Lysis →Anemia
Immune (Ab–Ag) Complex	• Inflammation • Opsonization • PMN Attraction & Activation	• Vasculitis • Serum Sickness
Anaphylaxis (IgE)	• Inflammation • ↑ Vascular Permeability • ↑ GI Secretion & Mobility • Expulsion of Inhaled Ag (?)	• Asthma • Anaphylaxis
CELLULAR		
Delayed-Type Hypersensitivity (esp. dermal)	• Intracellular Organisms • Viral Immunity	• Contact Dermatitis • Autoimmunity
Granulomas	• Isolated Organisms	• Tissue Destruction

Figure 3.3. Category Chart: Basics of Immune Responses

SOURCE: Figure provided by Kent R. Folsom, M.D., Harrisonburg Emergency Physicians, Harrisonburg, VA.

Cell	Origin/Location	Functions	Features/Morphology	Lifetime	Receptors
NEUTROPHIL (Polymorpho-Nucleocyte)	Bone Marrow → Circulation 3 Days ↓ Circ → Lungs, Spleen	**ACUTE** Inflammation: Phagocytosis Some in *Chronic* Inflamm.	1° (Azurophilic) & 2° Lysosomal Granules Amoeboid Motion	Short	Complement C3b; IgG – Fc
BASOPHIL		**ACUTE Allergic & Anaphylactic** Reactions (a Mast Cells) Discharge of Granules, 1° Histamine; Heparin & Eosinophil Chemotactic Factor	Basophilic Granules Lobated Nucleus		IgE – Fc
EOSINOPHIL		1° **Allergic,** Parisitic 2° *Chronic* Inflammation Antagonizes Basophils & Masts Kills Parasites	Granules & Major Basic Protein (Kills Parasites) Histaminase		

Figure 3.4a. Category Chart: Cell Types

SOURCE: Figure provided by Kent R. Folsom, M.D., Harrisonburg Emergency Physicians, Harrisonburg, VA.

Cell	Origin/Location	Functions	Features/Morphology	Lifetime	Receptors
MONOCYTES → Macrophage	Bone Marrow 3 Days → Random Entry into Tissue → Enlarge to Mφ	*Chronic* Inflammation: Phagocytosis, Hydrolysis of Ingested Particles (broader range than neutro) Process Antigen for Presentation to Helper T-Cells	Azurophilic Granules Can Coalesce To Form Giant Cells; Kidney-bean shaped nucleus; Large Amounts of Cytoplasm	2 weeks to years	C3b IgG – Fc
LYMPHOCYTE B, T → Plasma Cell		*Chronic* Inflammation Humoral & Cell-mediated Immunity; Immunologic & Non Imm. Inflammation Plastacell → Ig Production	Clumped Dark Chromatin; Non-specific Migration to Inflammation		None (Non-specific)

Figure 3.4b. Category Chart: Cell Types (continued)

Receptor	Fiber	Modality	Senses	Adapting	Skin	Encapsuled
Hair Follicle	Aβ Aδ	Tactile			Hairy	no
Meissner's Corpuscle	Aβ	Tactile	Low frequency flutter; velocity	Rapid	Glabrous	yes
Pacinian Corpuscle	Aβ	Tactile	High frequency; velocity	Rapid	Glabrous; Hairy	yes
Ruffini Corpuscle	Aβ	Tactile	Maintained stimulus	Slow	Glabrous; Hairy	yes
Merckel Receptor	Aβ	Tactile	Maintained Stimulus	Slow	Glabrous; Hairy	no (expanded)
Free Nerve Ending:						
Cold Receptor	C	Temperature	10°–30°C Temp; Above 45°C, Paradoxical Cold			No
Warm Receptor	C	Temperature	>30°C; Max. @ 45°C			No
Nociceptor	Aδ	Pain	High threshold; pinch, prick			No
	Aδ	Pain	Heat, Cold			No
	C Polymodal	Pain	Heat >45°C; Chemical, Noxious			No
	C	Pain	Mechanical, Cold			No

Figure 3.5. Category Chart: Skin Receptors

SOURCE: Figure provided by Kent R. Folsom, M.D., Harrisonburg Emergency Physicians, Harrisonburg, VA.

- Optimal number of categories for either a row (across) or a column (down) is about five to six. A bigger chart loses visual impact and can't be reviewed quickly.
- Aim for a chart that can be reviewed in less than five minutes. Remember, review = recalling to consciousness information you have already learned (comprehended).
- If the lecturer gives details that are not in the text, be sure these facts are in your chart.
- Always have a "Miscellaneous," "Etc.," "Other Facts," "Comments," or "Special Characteristics" column for details that do not fit the compare-and-contrast format of the rest of the chart.
- If there is only one detail in a column, eliminate the column and put this fact in your Miscellaneous or Other column, or see if you can organize the main heading to incorporate this fact (e.g., make it a different color).
- To be useful for review, your charts should condense information. Otherwise, you won't be able to go through them repeatedly. Topics differ: Some are easily condensed and you can get 15 to 20 pages on a chart; sometimes, only 5 pages of information makes a chart. But your goal is to *condense.*
- Make your charts as visually interesting as possible so that you'll remember them. To keep the number of categories lower, you can color code and/or group similar items.
- Whenever possible, organize the columns in some logical way, for example, start with "Mechanism of Action" for pharmacology charts, because the rest of the information will be related to that organizing principle. Start internal medicine charts with "Symptoms," because that's naturally the first piece of information you get in time sequence.
- Consider using Post-its for organizing tentative charts. You can then move the concepts and details around until you are satisfied with them. (Some students have said they do this on a large open space such as their walls or mirrors!)
- Charts can be used for regular review once or twice a week (repeated practice).
- Using charts developed by other students isn't as beneficial as using charts you've created for yourself (but are better than having fewer reviews!).

- What you have on your chart will be remembered—so be sure the facts on the chart are correct. It's harder to "unlearn" something learned incorrectly than to learn the correct information in the first place.
- Use your computer to make either templates or the charts themselves.
- Efficient charting saves time in the long run and can lead to better grades because charts are
  — organized,
  — condensed for repeated reviews,
  — formatted to permit self-testing.

Occasionally, students decide to divide the information presented in a course into sections, each taking responsibility for condensing and organizing their assigned portion. Then they share these among the group. The obvious advantage of this cooperative effort is saving time by splitting up the task, theoretically leaving more time for review and self-testing. But most students say they prefer to make their own charts, because grappling with the organization of the material and having to think about how the information is organized brings insights, and the struggle often embeds the information more deeply in memory. Relying on the thoroughness and completeness of the information collected by another person can be risky.

Advantages and Disadvantages

There are many advantages to the use of category charts. They force you to break down information into main ideas and details. They provide a logical context for association, which aids recall. Clustered information is easier to remember. They are easy to review, especially compared with rereading the 10 pages of text they may summarize. Category charts make it easy to test yourself over a large body of information. Because the details in the boxes will appear later on tests, most students find a way to cover the boxes with a blank paper or fold the chart while they self-test for recall.

Frankly, we can think of no disadvantages.

Flowcharts

Flowcharts are used for material that is logically ordered in a temporal sequence—for example, cycles in biochemistry, blood clotting cascade, progression of a disease, sequence of T-cell activation, and so on.

A flowchart begins at the top or side of the page with the first stage/step/event of a sequence with arrows or lines extending to the next step(s) in the sequence, ending with the final product or outcome of the process, sequence, or cycle. The detailed information is boxed along the flow of information.

If you have a computer, you may want to investigate using flowcharting software to create your charts.

The virtue of flowcharts is nicely illustrated by the actomyosin cycle chart shown in Figure 3.6. Events occur in sequence but can feed back in complex circular routes. This flowchart presents a clear visual image of conceptual material that might otherwise be difficult to explain. The chart could have been drawn with numbers in the boxes and explanations for each number on the reverse side for ease in self-testing.

Advantages and Disadvantages

An advantage of the flowchart is that it forces you to break down the components in a sequence. The visual representation of information makes it easier to review and remember. Flowcharts provide a logical context for organization, which aids recall and can be used for self-testing. To self-test, cover a portion of the chart with blank paper, then reproduce the covered part on the blank covering sheet. You can also quickly sketch out a flowchart during an exam and refer to it while answering questions.

Provided they are created in such a way that review and self-testing can easily take place, there are no real disadvantages to the use of flowcharts.

Diagrams

Diagrams are used where the name and location of a structure is the key issue—for example, gross anatomy or histology. The structure can be copied from a text or drawn freehand. The parts of the structure to be learned should be numbered. Lines can be drawn from the number to the margin where the structures are labeled or named. The marginal details can then be covered while self-testing.

There are excellent diagrams in gross anatomy textbooks. The problem is that you can't sort them. You could copy them and number the structures you need to know. Many students say, however, that the act of drawing the structure and labeling each part makes the information more memorable.

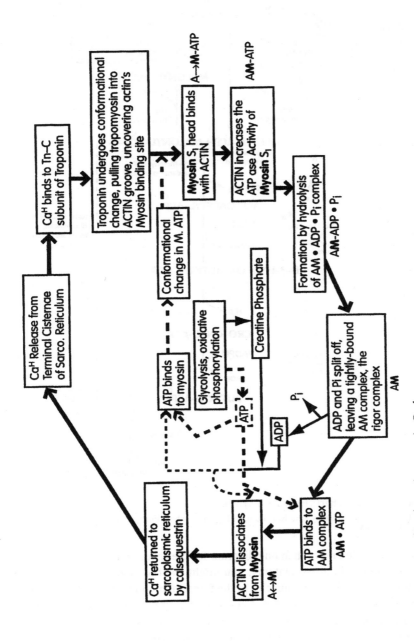

Figure 3.6. Flowchart: Actomyosin Cycle
SOURCE: Figure provided by Kent R. Folsom, M.D., Harrisonburg Emergency Physicians, Harrisonburg, VA.

71

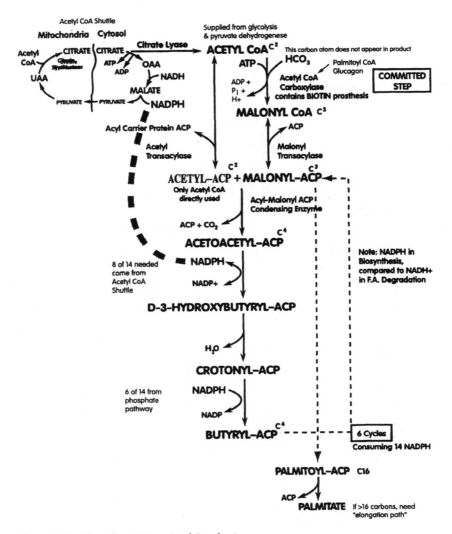

Figure 3.7. Flowchart: Fatty Acid Synthesis
SOURCE: Figure provided by Kent R. Folsom, M.D., Harrisonburg Emergency Physicians, Harrisonburg, VA.

You may need more than one diagram for the same structure. For example, on the forearm in gross anatomy, you might want to have separate diagrams for bones of the forearm, muscles of the forearm, blood vessels of the forearm, and nerves of the forearm. Draw lines from the numbered structures to the side margin where you can label each structure.

For a diagram, you can number the structures you need to know and create a key on a separate page. To self-test, number and letter a blank sheet of paper.

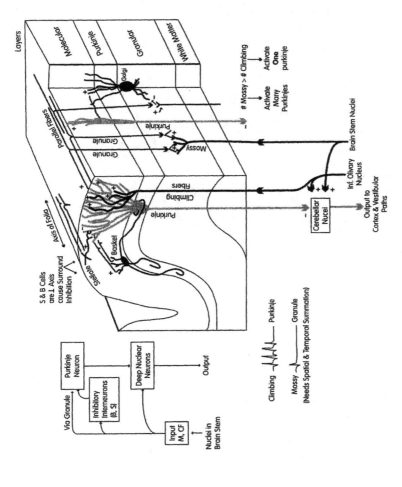

Figure 3.8. Diagram: Cerebellar Neuron Relationships
SOURCE: Figure provided by Kent R. Folsom, M.D., Harrisonburg Emergency Physicians, Harrisonburg, VA.

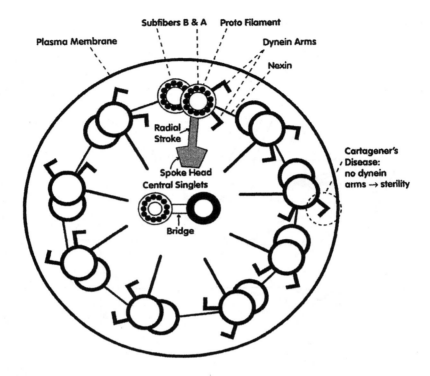

Figure 3.9. Diagram: Cilia Structure
SOURCE: Figure provided by Kent R. Folsom, M.D., Harrisonburg Emergency Physicians,
Harrisonburg, VA.

To self-test, the student would number and letter a blank sheet of paper and
fill it in from memory (covering the key to the diagram) and then check those
answers against the key. Actually writing down the answers and checking them
against the key eliminates the "Oh, that looks familiar, I must already know
that" phenomenon (which seems to produce surprisingly low test scores).

Advantages and Disadvantages

Diagrams are the logical way to make notes about structures. Their pictorial
quality makes them interesting and easy to remember. They can be constructed
with labels on the side for self-testing and therefore sorted into "know" and
"don't know" stacks, allowing you to focus your attention and giving you
further review time on what you don't know. You can redraw them on the
margins of a test paper, to recall the information during an examination.

There are no disadvantages to using diagrams as study notes, except that their use is limited to information for which knowledge of structure and the names of parts of a structure are important, such as in anatomy. For some courses, there will be little or no need for diagrams.

Combined Note Forms

Combined note forms can also be useful in many cases. The possible combinations are nearly endless, but we've chosen just a few to illustrate the possibilities. This is your chance to be creative!

The original cardiac physiology chart shown in Figure 3.10 was taped horizontally into one long chart. With the key on the second page, it is easy to self-test from.

Mapping

Mapping came to the attention of medical educators in the mid-1980s. There are several varieties of mapping strategies. Knowledge maps, concept maps, networking, and semantic maps are some of the more popular types.

Maps somewhat resemble flowcharts, except that they are not necessarily unidirectional. They are usually hierarchical, with the major topic at the top or center of the map. They deal with conceptual relationships, and the connections among themes may go in any direction.

Students in problem-based curricula are most likely to encounter mapping as a note-making strategy. It is possible to make a map of an entire discipline, for example, but information at the general conceptual level is not typically required on the objective examinations offered at most medical schools. Medical examinations tend to be very detail oriented. Maps are often associated with problem-oriented learning because they encourage students to cross traditional topic boundaries to seek relationships among information.

Advantages and Disadvantages

Maps are useful for describing what you already know about a subject. They can help improve the transfer of knowledge from one area or discipline to another, and teacher-created maps can be especially helpful in getting an overview of a topic or even a whole course.

However, mapping is an acquired skill, which can take several hours of training before you are able to use it. It is not necessarily intuitive. In general,

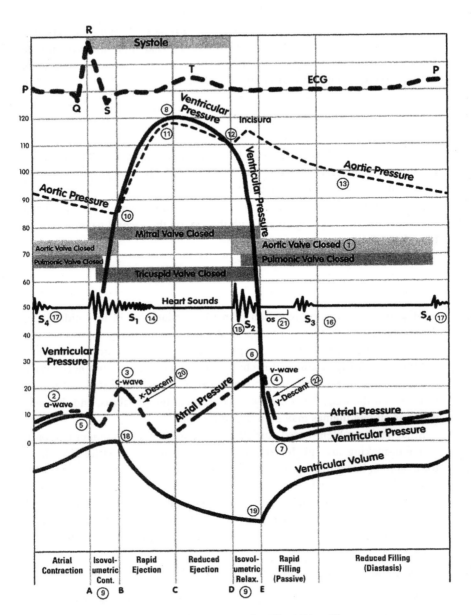

Figure 3.10a. Combined Note Form: Cardiac Physiology Chart

SOURCE: Figure provided by Kent R. Folsom, M.D., Harrisonburg Emergency Physicians, Harrisonburg, VA.

(1) Aortic valve closes due to elastic recoil of aorta

(2) a-wave due to pressure increase 2° to atrial contraction

(3) c-wave due to: (1) return of blood forced into pulmonary veins during atrial contraction and/or (2) mitral valve bulging into atrium when LV contracts

(4) V-wave occurs as blood that is filling LA from pulmonary circuit forces mitral valve open and blood rushes into LV

(5) Ventricular pressure recorded just before systole is the end-diastolic pressure coincident with R-wave of ECG

(6) Ventricular end-systolic pressure (also residual volume)

(7) Note wide R gap between LA & LV pressures ⇒ rapid filling. This effect of elastic recoil of LV muscle produces "negative" pressure with respect to LA

(8) Ventricular systolic pressure

(9) Isometric since both mitral & aortic valves are closed. Also "isovolumetric"

(10) Aorta valve opens as LV pressure exceeds aortic pressure. This is the diastolic blood pressure

(11) Aortic systolic pressure. This and #10 reflect the activity of the LV.

(12) Incisura is due to elastic recoil of aorta and arteries. Blood hurls back, slamming aortic valve leaflets

(13) Pressure decline is due to flow of blood into tissues. Pulsatile nature is absorbed by elasticity in aortic tree.

(14) Low-frequency/high amplitude component of S_1 is due to closure of A-V valves and the opening of the semilunar valves. The high-frequency/low amplitude component is due to turbulent flow (Reynold's number is exceeded) of blood into the aorta and pulmonary artery.

(15) S_2 is a short-duration/low-frequency sound caused by abrupt closure of the semilunar valves and the rebound of blood against them.

(16) S_3 (more prominent in children & adolescents) is due to vibrations of ventricular walls during rapid filling

(17) S_4 is due to ventricular vibration due to atrial contraction & blood influx

(18) End-diastolic volume is the maximum volume in heart prior to contraction

(19) End-systolic volume is the residual blood volume following contraction. The ejection fraction is stroke volume/end-diastolic volume; stroke volume is ESV-EDV

(20) Drop in pressure due to movement of the base inferiorly, expanding the atria. This is the **most visible** of the jugular pulsations. Descent & c-wave are artifacts of heart motion.

(21) Location of opening snap in mitral stenosis

(22) Drop in atrial pressure as A-V valves open and ventricles continue to expand (act as one big chamber)

Figure 3.10b. Cardiac Physiology Chart (continued)

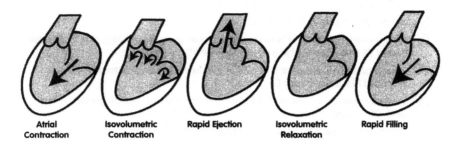

Atrial Contraction	Isovolumetric Contraction	Rapid Ejection	Isovolumetric Relaxation	Rapid Filling

Figure 3.10c. Cardiac Physiology Chart (continued)
SOURCE: Figure provided by Kent R. Folsom, M.D., Harrisonburg Emergency Physicians, Harrisonburg, VA.

mapping emphasizes main ideas over details, although some styles provide for elaboration of the overview in subsequent maps.

Self-testing would require you to re-create the map from memory—although some users of the mapping strategy report that the lack of inherent structure makes some maps difficult to re-create and mapping proponents discourage memorization of maps anyway. If you choose mapping as a note-making strategy, it is important to develop a system of review and self-testing that allows you to re-create the information you have stored in map form.

Figure 3.13 shows an example of a knowledge map created by a medical educator.

Why Not Outline?

You may have wondered why outlining as a form of note making has not been recommended, although teachers and many other study skills books go to a lot of trouble to teach you how to do it. Outlining is not as satisfactory for medical school study notes, because anything you can outline, you can put into category charts, which are better organized and more memorable.

- Category charts visually display the network of relationships among the details of the topic better than outlines.
- It's hard to self-test from an outline.
- Outlines don't work well for relationships involving cause and effect or temporal change.

a.

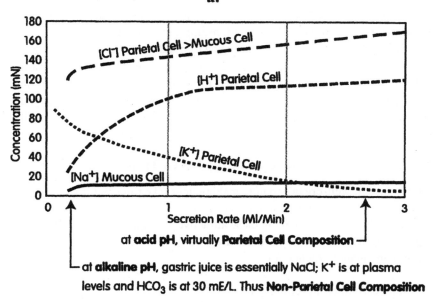

at **acid pH**, virtually **Parietal Cell Composition**

at **alkaline pH**, gastric juice is essentially NaCl; K^+ is at plasma levels and HCO_3 is at 30 mE/L. Thus **Non-Parietal Cell Composition**

b.

Condition	Representative Ranges	
	Basal Acid Output (mEq/hr)	**Maximal Acid Output (mEq/hr)**
Normal	1–5	6–40
Gastric Ulcer	0–3	1–20
Pernicious Anemia	0	0–10
Duodenal Ulcer	2–10	15–60
Zollinger-Ellison Syndr. (Gastrinoma)	10–30	30–80

Figures 3.11a and b. Combined Note Form: Rate and Composition of Gastric Acid

SOURCE: Figure provided by Kent R. Folsom, M.D., Harrisonburg Emergency Physicians, Harrisonburg, VA.

When students say they're outlining, they're often just making not very organized "loose notes." They don't consistently subordinate information in a hierarchical fashion or show relationships among the topics.

Reference to the category chart shown in Table 3.1 will help you decide how to choose the best type of note for your purpose. This table summarizes the different types of notes discussed in this chapter and, thus, nicely illustrates the usefulness of category charts. This "decision table" will help you to analyze the task first by asking yourself, "What kind of information is this?"

Note Making Takes Time

Let's face it, well-organized note making does take time, but it goes faster as you become proficient. Making notes is an active learning process. Plus, all the work you put into making these attractive and functional notes in the first place pays off repeatedly in future uses. You will have many opportunities to use them again to review for

- block/midterm/preliminary exams,
- final course exams,
- medical licensing examinations,
- clinical cases.

Storing Your Notes

Because you'll refer to these notes again and again, you'll need a good system for storing them and a way to quickly retrieve the ones you want.

Category and flowcharts can be filed either in tabbed three-ring binders or in file folders. You can buy file boxes designed especially for note cards (such as recipe boxes) to store your flash cards.

The bottom line in note making is this: If you can't make a set of condensed, organized notes, you don't understand the material. As soon as you see the relationships between the different bits of information, there should be no problem making your notes.

Exercise: Reading and Note Making

- Using one of the Time-Monitoring Worksheets from Chapter 1, add "RN" (for reading and note making) to the time you go back over the text and lecture notes to create your own set of condensed notes for review.

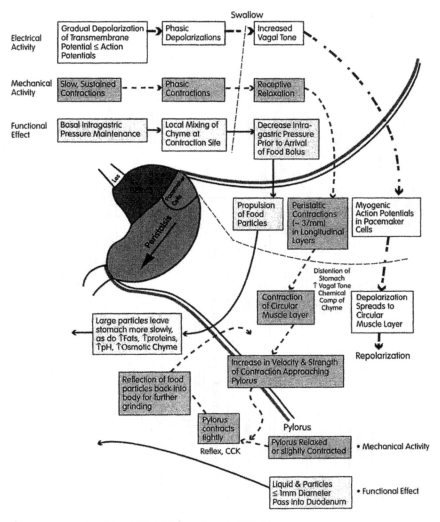

Figure 3.12. Combined Note Form: Gastric Motility

SOURCE: Figure provided by Kent R. Folsom, M.D., Harrisonburg Emergency Physicians, Harrisonburg, VA.

Note: Reading and note making will require 2 to 4 hours a day, five days a week and one long or two shorter study periods on the weekend—between 15 and 25 hours per week total. This will be your main study activity outside of lecture and lab. The time will vary, of course, depending on how quickly you are able to comprehend the material and organize your notes. A period of reading and note making includes combining information on that topic from your texts, note service notes, syllabus, and your own class notes into the one

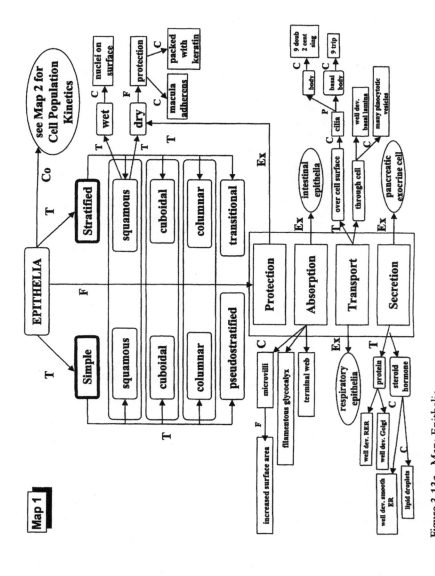

Figure 3.13a. Map: Epithelia
SOURCE: Map provided by Jennifer Peel, Ph.D., University of Arkansas Medical Sciences.

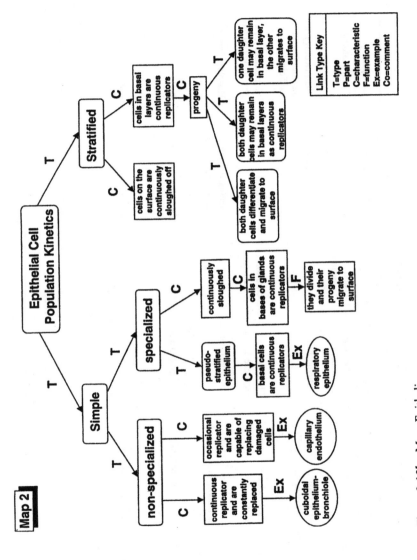

Figure 3.13b. Map: Epithelia
SOURCE: Map provided by Jennifer Peel, Ph.D., University of Arkansas Medical Sciences.

What to use for kinds of Info

Table 3.1 Decision Table: How to Choose the Best Note Making Format

If the Task Is to	And the Information Is	Make This Type of Note	Examples
Associate a name with a location	Static/unchanging and related information is due only to location	Diagram	Gross anatomy
Compare and contrast or classify a set of main topics according to a set of similar details	Static/unchanging	Category chart	Pharmacology, microbiology, diseases (e.g., pathology or internal medicine)
Associate a complicated series of names, procedures, or functions	Changing in a temporal chronological sequence or cause/effect sequence	Flowchart	Biochemistry, parasitic life cycles, physiology, or any process
Associate complicated but related set of information involving names, location, and details of function	Static/unchanging	Combine diagram with a category chart	Histology, neuroscience
Compare and contrast and see contacts between more than one complicated, but related, process	Changing in a temporal/chronological sequence	Combine flowchart by categories	Endocrinology
Recall unrelated, specific information (e.g., definitions or formulas); very small charts; or details from larger charts that you still need to learn	Not complicated enough to require a full 8½″ × 11″ sheet of paper	3″ × 5″ cards	Any class
To get the "big picture" of a topic at a conceptual level	Irregular, complex associations—including cause and effect	Map	Overview, across disciplines, whole systems

set of information that you will absolutely know. If it will be helpful, use one of the worksheets to monitor your reading and note-making time. Remember, the process will go faster the more you practice it.

- Decide what type of review notes (or combination) makes the most sense for each course you are taking. As you preview the course text and/or syllabus, your study notes, and any other material you've collected, make a mental note of what type of material it is (flowchart, category chart, etc.).
- If the topics you're studying include appropriate content, make at least one of each type of note this week.

☞ At the end of the week, return to this section and answer these questions.

Check-Up for Exercise: Reading and Note Making

1. In what way did you understand the material better after you made the notes?

_____

_____

_____

2. What types of notes did you make for each class?

_____

_____

_____

3. Does the information feel more familiar and more like it's "yours" now that you've worked with it?

_____

_____

_____

Students Say

"Making charts really helped me to concentrate my study materials into an amount I could review for the test."

"The note-making tips helped me look for what's important in a lecture."

"I used to waste study time not learning while reading. Now it takes less time to learn more, because I concentrate what I've studied into charts."

"I'm so glad I put forth the effort to make charts of my pathology notes in second year. I kept them in a separate notebook and used them a number of times throughout my junior year. I know I will continue to use my notebook frequently in my senior year and during my residency."

"I refer to my charts all the time."

"Some of my charts are so useful that I've condensed them further and carry them with me on the wards."

"I have referred to my charts from basic sciences during my clinical sciences rotations. I use them for a quick review before faculty rounds."

Summary

Creating a good set of notes for review and self-testing is the heart of the SWS system, but you cannot accomplish this unless/until you are scheduling solid blocks of time daily for reading and note making. Your notes will answer your questions about what, of all the information presented in lectures and texts, is important enough that you will be expected to know it not only on the next test but in the future in related courses and in clinical work. If you persist in making the kinds of notes described in this chapter, you will find that your thinking about information will become increasingly more organized. You will begin to see logical relationships between details and concepts more clearly in whatever you study.

If You Want to Know More

Annis, L. F., & Davis, K. J. (1977). Study technique and cognitive style: Their effect on recall and recognition. *Journal of Educational Research, 71,* 175-178.

Study indicates that underlining while reading leads to greater understanding than reading alone, but writing notes while reading is significantly better for retention than reading and highlighting.

Bretzing, B. H., & Kulhavey, R. W. (1979). Note-taking and depth of processing. *Contemporary Educational Psychology, 4*(2), 145-153.

Students who take notes on reading assignments perform better on exams, and the more reorganized their notes, the greater their comprehension and recall.

Brown, A. L., Compione, J. C., & Day, J. D. (1981). Learning to learn: On training students to learn from texts. *Educational Researcher, 10,* 14-21.

Describes the possible relationships among different types of information to be learned and the effect on learning of incorporating those relationships into notes.

Bruner, J. S. (1961). The act of discovery. *Harvard Educational Review, 31,* 21-32.

Demonstrates the importance to the learner of organizers in storage and recall. The act of making one's own system or organizers is the learning process.

Edmondson, K. M. (1994). Concept maps and the development of cases for problem-based learning. *Academic Medicine, 69,* 108-110.

Concept maps are often associated with problem-based learning because they encourage students to cross topic boundaries and disciplines to find relationships among information.

Holley, C. D., & Dansereau, D. F. (1984). Networking: The technique and the empirical evidence. In *Spatial learning strategies: Techniques, applications and related issues* (pp. 81-108). New York: Academic Press.

Describes the mapping strategy, called "networking," developed at Texas Christian University and discusses the theoretical basis for this strategy.

Isaacs, G. (1989). Lecture note-taking, learning and recall. *Medical Teacher, 11*(3/4), 295-302.

Review of literature on student note taking and the extent to which students actually learn as a direct or indirect result of taking notes.

Lambiotte, J. G., Dansereau, D. R., Cross, D. R., & Reynolds, S. B. (1989). Multi-relational semantic maps. *Educational Psychology Review, 1*(4), 331-367.

> *Describes features of knowledge maps and considers both their strengths and weaknesses.*

Novak J. D., & Gowin, D. B. (1984). Concept mapping for meaningful learning. In *Learning how to learn* (pp. 15-54). New York: Cambridge University Press.

> *This is the book that introduced concept mapping to medical educators. The authors discourage the memorization of maps.*

Peper, R. J., & Mayer, R. E. (1978). Note-taking as a generative activity. *Journal of Educational Psychology, 70*(4), 514-522.

> *Outlines three possible explanations for why the overt activity of note making affects the learning outcome: (a) increases overall attention and orientation to new material, (b) requires more effort and deeper encoding of the material than does merely reading, (c) requires organizing and "making sense" of the material, which tends to integrate new material to information acquired previously.*

Pinto, A. J., & Zeitz, H. J. (1997). Concept mapping: A strategy for promoting meaningful learning in medical education. *Medical Teacher, 19*(2), 114-121.

> *Discusses components of meaningful learning and proposes training in concept mapping to enhance learning.*

Polk, S. R. (1995). *Medical student's survival guide: Career strategy for changing times.* Myrtle Beach, SC: Trentland.

> *Pages 18-19 give a realistic view of trying to sip from the basic science fire hose of information but do not give advice on how to cope.*

Quirk, M. E. (1994). *How to learn and teach in medical school.* Springfield, IL: Charles C Thomas.

> *Although memorization is currently somewhat devalued in medical education, particularly in problem-based curricula, memory and thinking are inextricably linked. Memorized facts need to be placed in larger context to be readily generalized to a variety of applications.*

Riegelman, R. K., & Hirsch, R. P. (1996). *Studying a study and testing a test: How to read the health science literature.* Boston: Little, Brown.

> *A practical guide for efficient reading of health literature. Very good information but too detailed for most medical students' purposes.*

Russell, I. J., Caris, T. M., Harris, G. D., & Hendricson, W. D. (1983). Effects of three types of lecture notes on medical school achievement. *Journal of Medical Education, 58,* 627-636.

> *Study showed that medical students who had to make their own notes from lectures had better retention of lecture information than students who received detailed handouts for the same lectures and did not need to create their own notes. Conclusion: Making notes embeds information in memory.*

Schwenker, J. A., Krogull, S. R., Rudolph, J. S., & Simpson, D. E. (1989). *Mastering medical content: A workbook for entering medical students.* Milwaukee: Medical College of Wisconsin.

> *This is a guide to ease the transition to medical studies. It also offers methods for improving academic performance. Chapter 4 illustrates a variety of methods for condensing and reorganizing content material.*

Shimmerlik, S. M., & Nolan, J. D. (1976). Reorganization and recall of prose. *Journal of Educational Psychology, 68*(6), 779-786.

> *Reorganization of material leads to improved academic performance on free recall tests.*

Willey, M. S., & Jarecky, B. M. (1976). *Analysis and application of information.* Washington, DC: Howard University, College of Medicine.

> *How to use outlines and charts for memorizing information, complete with many examples.*

4 Reviewing and Self-Testing From Your Condensed Notes

(Week 3)

> **Student:** "I just don't understand why I got a D on the last test. I really knew that material."
>
> **Mentor:** "How do you *know* you knew the material?"
>
> **Student:** "Well . . . it all looked familiar to me."

Diagnose Yourself: Reviewing and Self-Testing

Directions: Circle the number that best describes your actual behavior during an academic term.

	Never	*Rarely*	*Sometimes*	*Often*	*Always*

(4) 3 2 1 0   1. There is so much information to review before exams that I can't get back over all of it.

(4) 3 2 1 0   2. I try to understand the general concepts instead of memorizing details.

0 1 2 3 (4)   3. I use my notes to test myself over each topic to be sure I know and can recall it.

0 1 2 (3) 4   4. I review all my notes (or highlighted or underlined passages) at least once a week for each class.

91

4 3 (2) 1 0   5. I don't have time to review my notes on a daily basis.

0 1 2 3 (4)   6. I am able to repeatedly review the material because I have
               put it into a highly organized form.

0 1 2 (3) 4   7. I identify the topics and details that don't stick in memory
               and focus my review time on them.

0 1 2 3 (4)   8. By the time I take the test over a body of information, I will
               have reviewed it at least twice and usually three times.

(4) 3 2 1 0   9. I don't know how well I know the material until I take the test.

___3૪___   **Total score** (sum of circled numbers)

☞ Stop.
Do not continue until you are
ready to score the assessment.

Scoring Directions: Reviewing and Self-Testing Diagnosis

Add up all the numbers you circled to find your overall score.

1. Condensing and organizing your notes properly will allow you to review
   the material repeatedly before an examination.

2. If you take objective exams, you will need to know details to answer the
   questions.

3. When you use your notes to test yourself over each topic, you can
   determine if there are any gaps in your knowledge that need to be filled
   by further review before the actual examination.

4. Reviewing is the secret to keeping the information you have learned thus
   far fresh in your memory and easy to recall.

5. You should make time to review your notes, because repeated review puts
   information into longer-term memory. Short daily review sessions enable
   you to have repeated reviews for all of your classes.

6. Being able to repeatedly review the material in a highly organized form
   greatly enhances your ability to remember that material.

7. It's a more efficient use of time to zero in on what you have not mastered.

8. Good. You should review the material several times before you are tested
   on it.

9. Waiting until you take a test is a little late to find out what you don't know! Self-testing will help you focus your study time on information you need to know *before* you take the exam.

Score Interpretation: Reviewing and Self-Testing Diagnosis

30-36—Very good!
23-29—Good but could use improvement
14-22—Need help
Below 14—Desperate need—*This chapter can really help!*

Once the notes are made, the hard part is done! You had to have some understanding of the information to make the notes; now you will just remind yourself of what you have determined you'll need to know.

Repetition is the key to memory.

Repetition is the key to memory.

Repetition is the key to memory.

Memory experts say distributed, or spaced, practice results in greater learning and longer retention of information than massed practice. Massed practice could also be defined as just one long study period, or cramming. Distributed practice ensures repetition. Repetition is known to increase retention and retard forgetting. Information that is repeated frequently is said to be "learned by heart" or "overlearned." Examples from everyday life are your Social Security number and frequently used telephone numbers or addresses. Typically, there are five to six weeks between exams for any one course. To review repeatedly, you should be caught up on all your note making by the end of every week. This allows you to review the information presented at the beginning of the course while you continue to accumulate new information and notes each subsequent week before the next exam. If you don't regularly review the material presented earlier in the period between tests, recently presented material pushes the older material further back in your memory, making it harder to retrieve. So how many repetitions can fit reasonably into a medical student's schedule? Ideally, you would review all the condensed notes you have made for each course once a week. Realistically, this probably won't happen. When nearing an examination, more time must be spent on the more recent material, because there is less time for repetition. Aim for at least two reviews of each set of notes, followed by two self-tests over the same material. Of course, if your self-test reveals that you do not know some particular information, you'll need to give those topics more review and self-testing. By the day of the test, you will have encountered the material at least seven times.

- First, you preread it before the lecture.
- Second, you heard it and took notes during the lecture.
- Third, you read the text carefully.
- Fourth, you created your condensed notes.
- Fifth, you did the minimum of one (preferably two or more) spaced review.
- Sixth, you did a minimum of one (preferably two or more) self-tests.
- Seventh, you did a quick overall review of all the topics before the exam.

Table 4.1 shows the Study Without Stress system at a glance.

Zeroing in on What You Don't Know

There are three good reasons to self-test, even if you're not a masochist.

- First, the alternative is waiting until the professor tests your knowledge. Tests are designed to let the teacher know if you have learned the information, but it's too late then for *you* to find out what you don't know.
- Second, you will save time. You will not have to focus as much attention on information your self-test reveals that you already have learned well and remembered. You can spend more time where you really need it: attending to that information you could not recall on your self-test.
- Third, self-testing gets your adrenaline flowing, raises your motivation to study and learn and focuses your attention.

It may be more emotionally satisfying to keep reviewing what you already know and to ignore what you don't know—but it's more **useful** to do the opposite!

Table 4.1 The Study Without Stress System at a Glance

Type of Study Activity	Approximate % of Time to Schedule	Approximate Amount of Time to Schedule	Time of Day/Week to Schedule	Purpose/Rationale for Study Activity	Study Behavior
Prereading	10	45 min-1 hour per day × 5 days per week 4-5 hours per week	Immediately prior to lecture or the evening before lecture	Advance organizer. See the big picture of the topic to be covered in lecture. Increase concentration during lecture. Get better lecture notes.	Use book or syllabus for abstract, summary, boldface words, italics, charts, diagrams, study questions. Ask yourself, "What is this page about?" or "What main topic is covered in this section/chapter?"
Reading and note making	70	3 hours per day × 5 days a week, plus an additional 5-6 hours on the weekend 20-21 hours per week	After lecture. Choose best time of day for high concentration. Schedule 2-3 hours consecutively if possible.	Fit details into the big picture. Understand how to apply principles, if appropriate. Organize into easily memorizable format, if a memory task. Make compact notes for review and self-test.	Undistracted concentration until you have a clear understanding of principles or of details and main topic. Make charts. Make diagrams. Make cards.
Reviewing	10	½ hour per day × 6 days per week 3 hours per week	Last study activity	Increase retention, speed, recall.	Reread charts, diagrams, cards—any condensed notes.
Self-testing	10	½ hour per day × 6 days per week 3 hours per week	When motivation drops during a study period or as a change from other study activities. At least weekly.	Increase motivation. Check on retention. Aid to planning further review of specific topics.	Sort flash cards. Cover details in charts and fill in details on another sheet of paper. Ask yourself questions and check the answers.

95

How to Self-Test

Note Cards

Note cards are good for memorizing details. Memorization may not be much admired as an intellectual pursuit these days; however, there are thousands of details to be remembered in medical science.

If you can answer the question on the cue side of the card, put the card in a "know" pile. If you can't answer the question, put the card in a "don't know" pile. Keep the "don't know" cards separate for further review. You can use rubber bands or clips to hold cards together in their "know" and "don't know" stacks.

Students report that they can really learn the 10 cards they carry with them each day. If you learn the 10 cards (or more) you carry six days each week, then during a 15-week semester, you will have learned nearly 1,000 bits of information during odd moments of time that would otherwise be completely lost!

Category Charts

Start self-testing after you have reviewed a chart twice. Self-testing increases motivation because it lets you know which details need more review. Put an "R" (for review) and "ST" (for self-test) on the bottom corner of each chart. Make a tally mark after the R each time you review and one after the ST each time you self-test.

There are at least two easy ways to self-test using category charts. The first one is to cover the inside boxes of the chart with a blank piece of paper, leaving the headings in the rows and columns uncovered. Reproduce the contents of the boxes by writing on the blank piece of paper used as a cover. If you do this both by rows (across) and columns (down), you will be certain you have all the comparisons and contrasts well embedded in your memory. Another method that students have found effective is to re-create the chart on a large whiteboard. The key is to *write* your answers so that you won't be tempted to fool yourself by saying, "That's what I meant," or, "Oh, I know that." If you really know it, you will be able to reproduce it.

Compared with 3" × 5" cards, category charts are harder to sort, but charts can also be sorted into "know" and "don't know" piles. It just takes longer, because there's so much more information on them. If only one detail that is not yet mastered keeps a chart from being sorted into the "know" pile, you can copy that detail onto a 3" × 5" card and carry it in your "10-a-day" stack until it's committed to memory.

Flowcharts

As with category charts, flowcharts are harder to sort into "know" and "don't know" piles than cards because they contain more information. But the same method would be used.

To self-test, cover the flowchart with a blank sheet of paper and re-create the flow in writing, uncovering it as you move down along the arrows. As with category charts, a whiteboard may be used instead of paper. The test is to accurately anticipate the next covered information in the sequence.

Diagrams

Self-testing with diagrams is accomplished by covering the marginal labels with a blank sheet of paper and writing the names of numbered or lettered structures on the covering paper. When all have been named, compare your covering sheet with the original labels. If you have mislabeled anything, sort that diagram into your "don't know" pile. Diagrams with everything correctly labeled by this method go into the "know" stack. As with other types of charts, single details may be copied onto 3" × 5" cards for further review.

Mapping

Self-testing would require one to re-create the map from memory, although this is discouraged by mapping experts. However, if you use mapping, it is our opinion that if it's important enough to map, you will need to review and practice re-creating it just as you would the other types of charts.

See Table 4.2 for a summary of uses of notes by type.

Tips for Reviewing and Self-Testing

- Keep track of reviews and self-tests by making tally marks on the charts or diagrams themselves. Review at least two times before self-testing.
- Consider using loose rings to hold your charts while reviewing and self-testing. You can easily combine and sort the charts as needed.

how to self-test

Table 4.2 Summary: Uses of Notes by Type

The following category chart summarizes how to use charts, diagrams, and cards both for review and self-test. See how useful category charts are?

Type of Chart	How to Self-Test	Advantages for Review and Self-Test	Disadvantages for Review and Self-Test	Storage
Category charts	Cover the inside boxes with a blank sheet of paper and see if you can duplicate the contents of the boxes in writing. Sort into "know" and "don't know" piles.	Can review quickly Easy to self-test	Harder to sort than cards Contain more information than cards	Filed in either tabbed 3-ring binders or in file folders
Flow charts	Cover labels in far margins and duplicate the answers in writing. Sort into "know" and "don't know" piles.	Easy to review Can be re-created from memory	Harder to sort than cards Contain more information than cards	Filed in either tabbed 3-ring binders or in file folders
Diagrams	Cover labels in far margins and duplicate the answers in writing. Sort into "know" and "don't know" piles.	Easy to review Can be re-created from memory	Harder to sort than cards Contain more information than cards	Filed in either tabbed 3-ring binders or in file folders
Note cards	Sort into "know" and "don't know" piles	Zero in on details not easily remembered	Lack of contextual/associational cues to memory	3″ × 5″ file box or band with a rubber band by topic

- Reviewing is *not* memorizing all at once. You *will* see this chart again. Do not spend more than five minutes per chart. You must get through *all* of them to ensure spaced practice.
- Understanding versus memorizing—You couldn't have made the chart or card in the first place if you didn't have some understanding of the material. Spaced practice means pulling it forward in your memory and registering it one more time.
- Using old classroom exams as a source of review can often be helpful. The important thing to remember is to look for *patterns* of errors; don't get hung up on any particular question. Keep in mind, too, that an old exam may not be representative of what will be on future exams. See Chapter 6 on test taking for a worksheet that will help you analyze test-taking errors.

When to Review and Self-Test

Weekends are ideal for reviewing and self-testing. This is probably the only time during the week you're not receiving new information. Use this time to catch up, review, and test yourself. About 30 minutes to an hour is what you'll spend on review each day. More, of course, just before an exam.

Study tip: Whenever you're in a reading and note-making study period and your mind begins to wander or you feel drowsy and are losing interest and motivation, it's time to self-test. You'll find out you don't know some piece of information. That will wake you up!

Exercise: Reviewing and Self-Testing

1. Carry 10 cards to review every day this week. Sort them at the end of each day. Carry the "don't knows" a second day, adding enough new cards to make 10 every day. Total the number of "know" cards at the end of the week.
2. Begin to review (and self-test after two or three reviews) and keep track of the number of reviews and self-tests by tallying them on the bottom corner of your charts, cards, or diagrams.

☞ **At the end of the week return to this section and complete the check-up below.**

Check-Up for Exercise: Reviewing and Self-Testing

- On the average, how many times a day were you able to sort through your stack of 10 cards?

  _____

- How many of the cards were you able to put in the "know" pile by the end of each day?

  _____

- In self-tests of the information on your charts and diagrams, were you able to pinpoint specific facts (or areas) that needed further review? What did you do with that information?

  _____

Students Say

"Now I know what I need to spend more time studying."

"I'm a confirmed card carrier!"

"I used my charts to prepare for board exams, too."

"I charted and printed up the whole pharmacology course. Now other students can use my charts for review."

"My charts were helpful as quick reviews during my clinical rotations. I was able to give better answers to some of the attendings' questions!"

Summary

As you began this book, you completed a number of exercises to ensure that you were scheduling enough time to study. You needed to do this, because your next step was to learn to make an organized, condensed set of notes. There are two principal reasons for making notes as we have recommended:

- They help you figure out what you need to know.
- They put what you need to know in a format that facilitates review and self-testing.

All of your previous effort (in creating these highly organized notes) was to give you the opportunity to conveniently review and self-test. This chapter shows you how to do that. You will understand the main principles from creating the notes, and the review and self-testing will ensure that you remember the details. These are the processes by which information is stored in long-term memory. Review and self-testing will also help you discover the details you don't know. You can then convert the unknown details into cards for further review. Review and self-testing are the reasons you made such careful notes in the first place.

If You Want to Know More

Colvin, R. H., & Taylor, D. D. (1978). Planning student work-study time in an objectives-based medical curriculum. *Journal of Medical Education, 53*, 393-396.

> *Authors calculate that a final review, "cramming," takes 1 hour for every 10 hours of reading and review.*

Corkill, A. J., Bruning, R. H., Glover, J. A., & Krug, D. (1988). Advance organizers: Retrieval context hypotheses. *Journal of Educational Psychology, 80*(3), 304-311.

> *Rereading notes had a significant effect on recall.*

Farr, M. J. (1987). *The long-term retention of knowledge and skills.* New York: Springer-Verlag.

> *A thorough review of the scientific literature on learning, memory, and retention.*

Jacobson, R. L. (1986, September 3). Memory experts' advice: Forget about that string around your finger. *Chronicle of Higher Education*, p. 49.

> *A survey of 68 psychologists actively involved in research on memory revealed their personal preference for writing things down as an aid to retention. In addition, they prefer organization and repeated review.*

Sisson, J. C., Swartz, R. D., & Wolf, F. M. (1992). Learning, retention and recall of clinical information. *Medical Education, 26,* 454-461.

Thirty-three medical students lost between 10% and 20% comprehension when taking the same test three months later with no review.

Spitzer, H. F. (1939). Studies in retention. *Journal of Educational Psychology, 30,* 641-656.

A study of forgetting before and after review shows significantly greater retention up to 60 days after reading, if the material is reviewed. Concludes that review should occupy 90% of study time, especially if the material is somewhat disconnected or detailed.

5 Concentration

(Week 4)

Student:	"I spend a lot of time studying, but I don't seem to get very far through the material. I keep falling behind. It's discouraging . . ."
Mentor:	"What keeps you from accomplishing your goals in your study time?"
Student:	"I don't know. I'll be sitting at my desk and reading my book and notes, and after a while I realize that I'm not thinking about my studies at all. Without being aware of it, I've been worrying for some time about financial problems. I'm wondering how I'm going to manage to pay this month's bills that are piling up."
Mentor:	"It's odd that your thoughts always digress to that topic. How does that happen?"
Student:	"Probably because the stack of unpaid bills are in a basket on the corner of my study desk."
Mentor:	"Ah, ha!"

Diagnose Yourself: Concentration Self-Assessment

Directions: Answer according to the following scale:

1 = *seldom* (0-20% of time)   2 = *sometimes* (21-40% of time)
3 = *regularly* (41-60% of time)   4 = *often* (61-80% of time)
5 = *almost always* (81-100% of time)

Write your answer on the line to the left of the number.

_4_ 1. I feel awake and alert during study periods.

_3_ 2. I study in a place free of noise or other distractions.

_4_ 3. Personal concerns do not interfere with my ability to concentrate.

_5_ 4. I study in a well-lighted workspace that is clear of books and papers that I am not using right then.

_5_ 5. I set minigoals for each study period, in terms of number of pages to read or notes to make or material to review.

_5_ 6. I make sure I'm "in the mood" when it's time to study.

_2_ 7. I do not study while reclining on a sofa or easy chair or in bed.

_2_ 8. I take "energizing" breaks (exercise, eating) to keep going during long periods of study.

_3_ 9. I do not feel sleepy or begin to doze while studying.

_5_ 10. I begin a study period with a positive thought about how much I intend to accomplish or how much interest I have in the information that I'll be studying.

_4_ 11. There are no background sounds or sights while I study.

_3_ 12. I do not daydream during study periods.

_5_ 13. I set specific goals to accomplish during a study period.

_2_ 14. I have a special place where I do most of my studying.

_4_ 15. When I begin to tire of one study activity—for example, reading and note taking—I switch to another study mode—review or self-testing.

_5_ 16. I do not stare vacantly (out the window, at the wall, or at the same page of text) during my study period.

_4_ 17. While studying, I do not wish I were doing something else.

_2_ 18. I study in a place devoid of my favorite things (food, music, magazines, posters, letters, photographs, souvenirs, etc.).

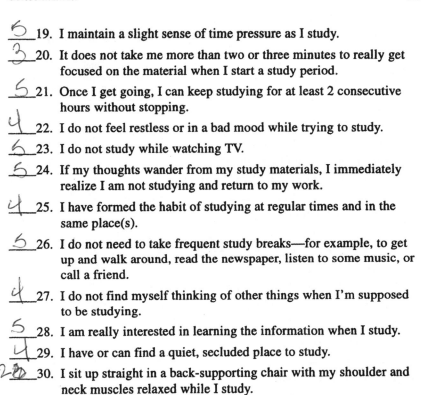

6 19. I maintain a slight sense of time pressure as I study.

3 20. It does not take me more than two or three minutes to really get focused on the material when I start a study period.

6 21. Once I get going, I can keep studying for at least 2 consecutive hours without stopping.

4 22. I do not feel restless or in a bad mood while trying to study.

6 23. I do not study while watching TV.

5 24. If my thoughts wander from my study materials, I immediately realize I am not studying and return to my work.

4 25. I have formed the habit of studying at regular times and in the same place(s).

5 26. I do not need to take frequent study breaks—for example, to get up and walk around, read the newspaper, listen to some music, or call a friend.

4 27. I do not find myself thinking of other things when I'm supposed to be studying.

5 28. I am really interested in learning the information when I study.

4 29. I have or can find a quiet, secluded place to study.

2 30. I sit up straight in a back-supporting chair with my shoulder and neck muscles relaxed while I study.

☞ **Stop.**
Do not continue until you are
ready to score the assessment.

Scoring Directions: Concentration Self-Assessment

Using the answers from the self-assessment, record the scores below for each of the items listed. Total the score across for each group.

Scoring Example:	My Score	Total Possible	My Percentage
1. Physically awake, alert			
Items: 1, 9, 16, 30			
Score: 4 + 4 + 3 + 2	= 13	÷ 20%	65

👉 *My Score ÷ Total Possible Points = My Percentage*

	My Score	Total Possible Points	My Percentage

1. Physically awake, alert

   1,   9,   16,   30

   $\underline{4} + \underline{3} + \underline{5} + \underline{2}$ = $\underline{14}$ ÷ 20 $\underline{70}$ %

2. Mood positive and under control

   6,   10,   17,   22,   28,

   $\underline{5} + \underline{5} + \underline{4} + \underline{4} + \underline{5}$ = $\underline{23}$ ÷ 25 $\underline{92}$ %

3. External distractions

   2,   4,   11,   18,   23,   29

   $\underline{3} + \underline{5} + \underline{4} + \underline{2} + \underline{5} + \underline{4}$ = $\underline{23}$ ÷ 30 $\underline{76}$ %

4. Internal distractions

   3,   12,   18,   24,   27

   $\underline{4} + \underline{5} + \underline{2} + \underline{5} + \underline{4}$ = $\underline{20}$ ÷ 25 $\underline{80}$ %

5. Work pace

   5,   13,   19

   $\underline{5} + \underline{5} + \underline{5}$ = $\underline{15}$ ÷ 15 $\underline{100}$ %

6. Discriminative stimuli

   7,   14,   20,   25

   $\underline{2} + \underline{2} + \underline{3} + \underline{4}$ = $\underline{11}$ ÷ 20 $\underline{55}$ %

7. Endurance for long periods of study

   8,   15,   21,   26

   $\underline{2} + \underline{4} + \underline{5} + \underline{5}$ = $\underline{16}$ ÷ 20 $\underline{80}$ %

(NOTE: #18 is both external and internal because the external stimuli may cue
   daydreaming or worrying.)

Score Interpretation:
Concentration Self-Assessment

Look back at the "My Percentage" column in each of the seven
categories above. (This number is derived from dividing your score
by the total possible points on each question.) Rank the *lowest*
percentage as your Number 1 concentration improvement priority,
the next lowest as Number 2, and the third lowest as Number 3.
Each of the seven categories will be discussed in the next section.
There are good enhancers to the SWS system in all seven categories,

but you will want to pay the most careful attention to your number 1, 2, and 3 priority categories and be sure to do the recommended exercises for them.

If none of your percentages were below 80%, congratulations! You may skip this chapter, if you'd like.

More Concentration = Less Study Time

It is often said that 80% of results are achieved in 20% of the time devoted to the task—the time a worker is highly focused and concentrating on the task.

No student is 100% efficient in the use of every hour of study time, but most students probably pay close attention 65% to 70% of the time. It is possible to raise the average rate of concentration closer to at least 80% by analyzing what is disturbing your study or slowing you down and eliminating some of that disturbance.

If you can increase the amount of serious concentration by 10%, you can gain about three extra hours of good study time each week. That may not sound like much, but over a semester, that would amount to an additional whole week (40-45 hours) of personal study time!

Seven Factors Affecting Concentration

To save time, first read the concentration factors you identified as your highest priorities. Do all the exercises for those factors. Then you have the option to read about the other factors and do those that seem most useful. All the advice and recommendations in this chapter can be used to improve your concentration and, thus, efficient use of time.

1. Alive, Alert, Awake

Feeling alive, awake, and alert improves any endeavor. It's hard to concentrate when your body is telling you it needs something: sleep, food, or exercise. Medical students, like athletes, need to keep themselves in good condition to perform.

Depriving yourself of bodily needs does not pay. In the short run, you lose concentration when your body is uncomfortable. In the long run, you may lose time due to illness. As a hard-working student, you need to sleep at least seven hours on weeknights with some extra sleep possible on the weekends. You also need to eat three decent meals a day and get some form of regular exercise, preferably on a daily basis. Fatigue, hunger, and muscular tension all interfere with studying. Although some students claim to be able to study into the wee hours of the morning, a careful analysis will most likely reveal that concentration drops after midnight or is very low in early morning classes.

Your bodily posture can affect your sense of physical alertness. If you are slumping or reclining while studying, the kinesthetic message is that you are resting or relaxing. Sitting up with a straight spine, feet flat on the floor, eyes on your work, and hands ready to manipulate your study materials tells your body that you are serious about what you are doing.

Exercise 1

Check your posture every 10 minutes during study sessions. Be sure that your feet are flat on the floor, your back is straight, and your eyes are directly over your work. If you are reading, follow the text down the page with your hand or a note card.

Exercise 2

Prepare energizing study break snacks in advance. We recommend vegetable sticks, cheese and crackers, nuts, or fruits. There is little or no preparation time with these snacks, and they boost energy quickly for the next round of study. Snack breaks should be taken in the 10-minute break between 50-minute study periods.

Exercise 3

Switch study activities when you begin to "phase out." Change to prereading (a brief activity anyway) or to review. When all else fails to rouse you from your lethargy, switch to self-test. Self-testing increases motivation, because you will discover what you don't know. Finding out what you don't know is a real "waker-upper."

Exercise 4

If you're sleepy or physically tired, do some vigorous exercise during your study break. Push-ups, toe touches, deep knee bends, jumping jacks, stretches—anything that will pump more oxygenated blood to your brain.

2. External Distractions

External distractions are a major problem, especially trying to study with music or television playing in the background. Many students deliberately turn on such noise and claim that it is not a distraction but rather an aid to studying. In your previous studies in college or high school, you did not need to maintain as high a level of concentration to cover the required information. If you currently tend to have music or TV in the background, ask yourself, "If I can hear and understand the music, radio voices, or television program, is not some part of my brain tracking that auditory and/or visual input while the other part is trying to study?" If you are getting any recognizable sensory signal from the background, it *must* be a distraction. If you can see or hear the potential distraction at all, turn it off. If it is not your intention to listen to or watch this sensory input, then it doesn't make sense to have it on.

Electronic devices aren't the only distractions students create for themselves. Some place their desks or study tables at a window where, whenever they look up from their books and notes, they can see outdoors. The view is an invitation to daydream and let your mind wander off your work to thoughts of the weather, people or vehicles passing by, what you might be doing if you were outside, and so on. Students also often surround their workspaces with photos of friends and family, souvenirs of special occasions, and other paraphernalia calculated to tempt their thoughts away from their studies. Do not let your eyes rove around the room or out the window.

It is possible to study in distracting conditions, but it takes more mental energy, leads more quickly to fatigue, and raises the odds that you will take longer to learn less.

Exercise 1

Clear the decks! Eliminate all distractions from your workspace. Place your desk or worktable against a blank wall. Have nothing on the work surface but the study materials for the *one class* you plan to study during that period. Keep books and notes from other classes on a shelf or table you can't see. This will prevent your thinking about what you should be doing for another class instead of concentrating on the one you have scheduled for that study time. When you have work for more than one subject in front of you, it's easier to feel ambivalent about what you should be doing and to vacillate from one subject to another.

Exercise 2

Make it hard to see anything but your work. If you have a very good lamp over your workspace, you can turn off any other lights in the room and you will see only what is directly in front of you. The light shining on the particular books and papers you are studying sharply focuses your attention on them and nothing else. Pretend that your eyes are a camera or microscope looking directly at the work in front of you.

3. Internal Distractions

Internal distractions are sometimes cued by external stimuli. The photograph of a special friend may make you start wishing you were at the beach having fun with him or her. External stimuli that pull thoughts away from your immediate task may be cued by

- piles of unpaid bills,
- stacks of unanswered correspondence,
- lists of things to do,
- unfinished household chores.

Cleaning the toilet can look very attractive when you're having difficulty convincing yourself that studying is what you want to do right now.

Worry is a potent internal distraction. And there can be plenty to worry about. Medical students have their share of relationship problems, family problems, and financial problems. Medical students are at an age when it is natural to be seeking companionship and thinking about a long-term relationship, if they do not already have a partner. After being in school almost all of their lives and not being able to earn much income, or returning to school after holding a full-time job, financial problems are fairly common. Parents of medical students may be dealing with some of the emotional and/or health problems of aging. Any or all of these concerns can become very severe and persistently force themselves into conscious thought.

Thinking about personal problems can ruin study time. It is essential that study time be devoted to study and nothing but study. This is your scheduled time to study today. This time will never come again.

So, what can you do?

Exercise 1

Keep a slip of scratch paper on your desk or table and make a note or check mark every time you find your mind wandering from the study materials in front of you. Also write down where your thoughts went. It's sometimes very surprising to what unimportant or trivial pursuits the mind can wander when out of control.

If your thoughts keep returning to a really serious problem that deserves your attention, get out your schedule and reserve a time when you are not scheduled for study to think about this problem.

Whatever you do, do not rob yourself of your study time. If the problem is not in your power to solve (and it's amazing how many of our worries fall into this category), you will find that you won't even use the scheduled "worry" time. Worrying is circular thinking that returns to the same point where it began, and usually your mind won't really want to do it according to a planned schedule. Problem solving is quite another matter. If it is a problem over which you have some control and is something you can resolve, you will find that time scheduled to decide your course of action is worthwhile. Just knowing that you have set aside a definite time to mull over this problem frees you to return to the task at hand, which is studying.

Exercise 2

Some students have used the following method to get rid of unwanted thoughts that creep in unaware while studying. Wear a rubber band on your wrist. As soon as you catch your mind wandering off the topic, "pop" the rubber band against your skin. This is what psychologists would call a mild "punishment." It is designed to extinguish undesirable behavior. It shouldn't really hurt; it's just to remind you to stop distracting yourself.

Exercise 3

If you catch yourself daydreaming, try this exercise. Close your book. Put down your pencil. Put away your papers. Then confront yourself about wasting your time. You can actually have a dialogue or argument with yourself. Remind yourself how important, even sacred, your study time must be if you are to achieve your goals. Tell yourself how useless it is to daydream when you should be studying. Don't let an open book give you the sense that you are working if you are not paying attention to the material. Vigorously remind yourself of what you want to accomplish during this study period. If you are alone (and therefore won't look crazy to someone else), argue out loud with yourself. Or you can write on a piece of paper all your counterarguments to whatever is the disruptive thought. Don't return to your studies unless/until you are sure you have your thoughts under control and can focus on your work.

4. Work Pace

It's easier to keep focused when you are working as fast as you can. When you dawdle over your work, unwanted thoughts or distractions are more likely to occur. For example, a sprinter running the 100-meter dash is not worrying about the menu for dinner that night. It's impossible to think of anything else while speed-reading. Adding the element of speed can make almost any task more exciting.

Exercise 1

Keep a sense of urgency while you study by setting a time limit to complete a task. Before you begin reading a textbook, decide how long it takes to read one page quickly. You need to make this experiment first, because some texts are more difficult or dense with information and will take longer to read. Multiply the number of minutes it takes to read one page quickly by the number of pages you plan to read during the next specific time period. For example, if you can read one page in five minutes, you can probably read six pages in 30 minutes. Make that your goal. This exercise creates a slight tension, which ensures that you keep working at your full capacity.

Exercise 2

Set yourself the goal of creating a set of organized notes over a specific topic within a limited time. For example, during one long concentrated period of study, set the goal of collating information on a particular topic and putting it into a set of cards, diagrams, or charts. You'll find yourself checking your watch and hurrying along to achieve the goal—and you won't find yourself daydreaming or nodding off to sleep.

5. Discriminative Stimuli

A discriminative stimulus is something in the environment that is a cue for an action or thought. A specific environment (study corner, desk, time of day) may be a discriminative stimulus for studying, whereas another environment (bed, sofa) is a cue for sleeping or relaxing. Actually, trying to study in bed can not only interfere with study and concentration, it can also be a cause of sleeping problems. Separate study from other activities. Also, if you schedule regular times for studying, it makes the stimulus stronger, just as certain times of day cue eating, sometimes even if you aren't especially hungry. Time as well as place can cue studying.

If you make good use of the stimulating power of objects, place, and time, you will be able to "get into" your work much faster, thus saving valuable time.

Exercise 1

If you do not have a special place to study, where you do nothing else but study, set up such a spot, preferably where you live. It can be as simple as a table, a lamp, and a chair. The simpler the better, to exclude distracting external stimuli. For between-class studying on campus, look for a quiet, out-of-the-way place in the library or an empty classroom, where you are not likely to chat with friends.

6. Mood Control

You can control your mood. Use emotion to help rather than hinder your study system. Setting the proper mood is the exact opposite of internal distractions.

Decide what internal messages work best to make you jump right into the task with a good will. It does no good to tell yourself something you can't believe, so be certain that your self-motivating talk is true for you. What may help you to think of valid self-talk is to recall what motivated you to apply to medical school in the first place. If you truly want to be a health professional, don't you really want to learn the information necessary to achieve that goal? Wouldn't you, in the long run, feel more satisfied having a clearer knowledge of how lipids metabolize (or any other study topic) than spending an hour daydreaming? You have decided on a career path that will always require you to work hard and concentrate your thoughts and physical energy on the task at hand. Lives may depend on your doing just that. You will be more fulfilled and work more efficiently if you keep reminding yourself that you really want to master this material.

Exercise 1

"Psych up" before you start a scheduled study period by saying something positive to yourself about studying and about the topic you are learning. You can establish a good mental set for concentration and focused study by vigorously repeating to yourself a variety of positive suggestions. For example:

"I really want to concentrate and get the most out of this time. I have everything I need to really learn about (name of subject) now. (The topic) is interesting and important to me. I am going to pay close attention to discover what is basic to understanding (this topic) well. I will also pay attention to significant details that contribute to understanding how the (main topic) works. I am going to focus all my thoughts on this topic. I'll keep my eyes fixed on the study materials. I'll see only my study materials. I really want to learn as much as I can about (the topic) right now."

7. Endurance

Endurance for long periods of study is increased with practice. High school students may consider an hour of study to be a lot of work. College students usually can work for a couple of hours and maintain a modicum of concentration. In medical school, you will probably need to schedule three or more sequential hours for highly concentrated study. You can, and probably should, take a 10-minute break at the end of each 50-minute study period. It's also a good idea to plan an entirely different activity at either end of a long period of concentrated study. If you keep yourself physically awake and mentally alert, eliminate both external and internal distractions, work at as fast a pace as the study topic permits, use discriminative stimuli to cue studying, and maintain a positive attitude toward your work, you will find that you can concentrate better for longer periods of time.

Exercise 1

After you've studied in a highly concentrated manner for several hours, reward yourself. Tell yourself how pleased you are with what you have accomplished. Admire your notes. Think about how much you have learned. Enjoy your break and know you deserve it.

Improve Your Concentration

For most students, lack of concentration is not the major weakness in their study system. But for those who do find lack of concentration to be a serious problem, the following exercise will help develop the habit of concentration and a keener awareness of your level of concentration.

Exercise: Record Concentration for One Week

If you find concentration to be a major problem for you—that is, you are not able to fully concentrate 80% of the study time—you should complete a week of concentration monitoring and answer all the check-up questions below. This assessment of your concentration levels will help you develop the habit of concentration and a keener awareness of your level of attention while studying.

Instructions:

- Tear out the Concentration Monitoring Timesheet (Table 5.1).
- Mark only your personal study time (in blocks of one or more hours) for each day.
- After each hour that you actually spend studying, mark (in the box immediately adjacent to the time) the level of concentration for that period. Estimate the percentage of time you maintain a good level of concentration according to the following scale.

1 = less than 20% of the hour   2 = between 21-40% of the hour
3 = between 41-60% of the hour   4 = between 61-80% of the hour
5 = between 81-100% of the hour

- Do this every day for one week.

☞ At the end of the week, return to this section and answer these questions.

Check-Up for Exercise: Record Concentration for One Week

1. What was your average percentage of concentration for each day?

   Monday _____ Tuesday _____ Wednesday _____
   Thursday_____ Friday _____ Saturday _____ Sunday _____

2. Was there a pattern to your concentration—that is, do you concentrate better at certain times of the day or best at the beginning, middle, or end of a period of study? Check your concentration monitoring sheet and note any patterns below:

   _____

   _____

   _____

3. When your concentration dropped during a study period, what was the cause?

   _____ Thinking of someone important in your life
   _____ Thinking of other obligations
   _____ Worrying about something
   _____ Thinking of other activities
   _____ Noises (TV, radio, stereo, roommate)

_____ The place you studied (library vs. home)
_____ Other—Please specify:

_____

_____

4. What can you do to avoid this disruption of your concentration?
_____ Clear your workspace
_____ Study in another place
_____ Schedule a special time to deal with the issue
_____ Assert yourself
_____ Wear ear plugs
_____ Other—Please specify:

_____

_____

_____

5. Having identified your patterns for concentration and its disruption, what
   do you need to do to ensure you get the most out of your study time?

_____

_____

_____

Students Say

Comments made **before** improving concentration exercises:

"I seem to put in enough hours of study time, but I don't feel I use the
time to my best advantage."

"I waste a great deal of time during my allotted study time due to lack of
concentration. I study only at about 70% concentration."

"I study 77 hours a week, but not all are quality hours."

Table 5.1 Concentration Monitoring Timesheet

Keep track of your study activities in half-hour or one-hour units for one week. Record major study activities using the following categories: LEC (lecture), LAB (laboratory), SLA (scheduled learning activities—e.g., seminars, review sessions), PR (prereading), RNM (reading and note making), and RVST (review and self-testing). **Estimate the percentage of your concentration during each of these activities.**

Name _____

Week of _____

	Monday		Tuesday		Wednesday		Thursday		Friday		Saturday		Sunday	
	Activity	% Conc	Activity	% Conc	Activity	% Conc	Activity	% Conc	Activity	% Conc	Activity	% Conc	Activity	% Conc
5:30 a.m.														
6:00														
6:30														
7:00														
7:30														
8:00														
9:00														
10:00														
11:00														
12:00 p.m.														
12:30														
1:00														
2:00														

| 3:00 |
| 4:00 |
| 5:00 |
| 5:30 |
| 6:00 |
| 6:30 |
| 7:00 |
| 7:30 |
| 8:00 |
| 8:30 |
| 9:00 |
| 9:30 |
| 10:00 |
| 10:30 |
| 11:00 |
| 11:30 |
| 12:00 |
| 12:30 |
| 1:00 |
| 1:30 |
| 2:00 |

Comments made **after** completing concentration exercises:

"I now make sure I am both physically and mentally prepared to study, and that's increased my concentration and self-confidence."

"Just clearing my study area has really helped me concentrate. I used to be overwhelmed by thinking of all the other subjects I should be studying, too!"

"Clearing everything off my desk has increased my reading speed by 100 words per minute!"

Summary

Students who have compared their level of concentration before and after completing the exercises in this chapter tend to find their "before" level of concentration between 60% and 70%. Their "after" level of concentration is closer to 80% or 85%. These exercises will help you stay "on task" during scheduled study periods. Over a 15-week term, a 10% gain in concentration would amount to 40 to 45 hours of otherwise wasted study time.

If You Want to Know More

Baker, R. W., & Madell, T. (1965). Susceptibility to distraction in academically underachieving male college students. *Journal of Consulting Psychology, 29,* 173-177.

Underachieving college students are more susceptible to distraction when studying—for example, conversations or background noise.

Collins, K. W., Dansereau, D. F., Garland, J. C., Holley, C. D., & McDonald B. A. (1981). Control of concentration during academic tasks. *Journal of Educational Psychology, 73,* 122-128.

Positive self-talk was found to enhance comprehension and retention of textual material.

Gibbs, J. J. (1990). *Dancing with your books: The Zen way of studying.* New York: Penguin.

Applies Zen methodology to attaining positive concentration during study.

Oetting, E. (1964). Hypnosis and concentration in study. *American Journal of Clinical Hypnosis, 7*(1), 148-151.

> *Research study shows hypnosis can improve study concentration. Gives examples of hypnotic suggestions that could be used by the student.*

Robinson, F. P. (1970). *Effective study.* New York: Harper & Row.

> *See the chapter on importance of concentration with some suggestions to improve it.*

Talley, J. E., & Henning, L. H. (1981). *Study skills.* Springfield, IL: Charles C Thomas.

> *Chapter on importance of concentration in study with specific suggestions on how to control daydreaming during study periods.*

6 Test-Taking Strategies

Diagnose Yourself: Test-Taking Strategies

Directions: Indicate whether each of the following statements is true or false in describing your test-taking behavior by circling T if true or F if false.

T F   1. During a test, I am disturbed by other students in the room.

T F   2. As soon as I am handed my test, I start answering the questions and work straight through the test, taking each one in numerical order.

T F   3. I usually leave the testing room early, before the full test time has elapsed.

T F   4. I answer every question if there is no penalty for guessing.

T F   5. I read each option on a multiple-choice question and consider each option as a separate question.

T F   6. I think about how many questions I have already missed as I work my way through a test.

T F   7. I sometimes return to test questions I've already answered and change them on the hunch I was wrong the first time.

T 8. In considering whether a multiple-choice option is true or false, I try to think of unusual exceptions or special cases.

T 9. I often "pull an all-nighter" before an exam.

T  10. I arrive early for exams and quiz my classmates, or have them quiz me, until the exam starts.

F 11. I underline key words in the stem of the question before choosing an answer.

F 12. Before starting to answer any questions, I calculate how much time is available for each test item.

F 13. I make a special note when a test item is negatively worded (e.g., uses the words "not" or "except").

F 14. If I don't see the correct answer immediately, I write what I do know about the topic on the test margin to look for a possible hidden relationship between the information I can recall and the response options available.

F 15. If I have to guess, I look for clues in the stem and options to indicate a possible best guess.

F 16. When the test time is up, I fill in answers on test items I don't have time to even read.

F 17. When I get back a scored test, I check it over to see the reasons I did not give correct answers.

F 18. I use all the time allowed for a test.

F 19. I know when it's a good idea to guess at answers I don't know from knowledge of content.

F 20. I answer all the easy questions first.

T  21. If the test lasts 60 minutes, and there are 40 questions, I spend a full 1½ minutes on each question.

T  22. My eating habits change greatly on the day or two before a major test.

 23. I live on caffeine for the day or so before a major test.

T F 24. I get stuck on one question and spend a long time trying to figure out the answer to it.

T F 25. I sometimes run out of time on tests.

☞ **Stop.**
**Do not continue until you are ready
to score the test-taking assessment.**

Scoring Directions: Test-Taking Diagnosis

Compare your answers on the test-taking assessment with the following correct answers. Give yourself 1 point for each answer you answered correctly.

1. **False.** If you are disturbed by others in the room during a test, you need to work on your concentration. Get earplugs or find the least distracting place in the room to sit during the exam. ✓

2. **False.** Answer all the easy questions first. Then go back and work over the harder questions. (See Number 14.) ✓

3. **False.** Use extra time to double-check your coding of responses on the answer sheet. Make sure you marked your answers in the right place on the response sheet. Go back and review any questions for which you had to guess to see if you have gained information later in the test to make a better choice or if you have a new insight. If not, do not change the answer! ✓

4. **True.** Guess when all else fails. There is usually no penalty for guessing either on classroom or standardized exams. The instructions will inform you if points are subtracted for wrong answers. ✓

5. **True.** Each option is a true-false question by itself and should be so considered. ✓

6. **False.** Thinking about how many questions you may have already missed makes you overanxious and interferes with your concentration. Save any such analysis for after you've completed the whole exam and are ready to turn it in. ✓

7. **False.** Research on changing answers indicates that first responses tend to be correct, so don't change an answer unless you have some new insight or recall some specific information that you didn't have in mind during your initial response. ✓

8. We hope you marked **false.** Remember, you want to give the "best" answer, not the "perfect" answer. Most truths have occasional exceptions, but that's not usually what is being asked in the question. ✓

9. **False,** or, at least, you shouldn't stay up all night before an exam. You won't be in optimal physical condition to take the test, if you do. ✓

10. **False.** If you marked true, consider that you are not likely to learn anything important at this stage and that you run the risk of making yourself overly anxious. ✓

11. **True.** Many a multiple-choice question has been missed by overlooking one key word in either the stem or a response option. ✓

12. **True.** At least, know where you want to be at one quarter, one half, and three quarters of the time allowed to complete the test.

13. **True.** Circle or double underline the word in the stem (e.g., *not, except, false*) that makes the item negative or reversed so that you won't forget it.

14. **True.** If you have time, you should list, chart, or draw a diagram in the test margin of what you can recall that is related to the question. This sometimes reveals connections not previously noticed.

15. **True.** There may be clues—such as length of an option, grammatical inconsistency, absolute words, qualifying words, similar options, absurd options, or word repetitions—that indicate a better guess.

16. **True.** Not having enough time doesn't usually happen on classroom tests but sometimes occurs on board exams. If you find yourself in the position of having to "dot in" many answers to items you don't have time to read, the best strategy, from a statistical point of view, is to select one column and fill in the dots straight down that column.

17. **True.** It's a good idea to review returned exams to discover the types of errors you made.

18. **True.** You should use all the time allowed. If time remains after you have marked all your answers, go back over the items to make sure you read them correctly and review your responses.

19. **True.** Guess whenever there is no penalty for guessing.

20. **True.** It's an excellent idea to go quickly through a test and answer the easy questions first, thus leaving more time for the harder ones.

21. **False.** Your calculation for the amount of time to give for each question should include a few minutes for review at the end or to go back and answer the hard questions you left blank.

22. **False.** It's not a good idea to drastically change your eating habits prior to an exam; you might not feel well physically during your final review or while taking the test.

23. **False.** Students have been known to be too sick to take a test because of overdosing on caffeine and not eating properly prior to a test.

24. **False.** If you spend too much time on a hard question, you risk not having time to get to other questions that you will be able to answer more easily. Better to make a mark in the margin next to this difficult item and come back to it after you have answered all the easier questions.

25. **False.** If you glance over the whole test before you start answering any questions and calculate how much time you have to spend on each one, this shouldn't happen.

Score Interpretation: Test-Taking Diagnosis

Read the section in this chapter concerning any topic you answered incorrectly.

20-25 = Good test-taking skills. Skim the chapter for additional tips.

15-19 = You're probably losing points on tests due to test taking errors. Read on!

Below 15 = Read this chapter carefully!

Why Tests Are Important

Most students measure their lives from one test to the next—either preparing for a test or recovering from one—and often say, "I live from test to test." And there are a great many tests. On average, during the basic sciences years, you will have at least four classes per term. In each class, there will probably be two or three midterms and a final. That's at least 12 major tests in each semester. If the midterms carry a lot of weight, any of these 12 or more tests can be crucial to passing the course. Almost all medical schools insist that every course be passed before a student can progress to the next term. Then there are the national board examinations. Many medical schools do not permit students to pass from the basic sciences to clinical studies until they have successfully completed the USMLE (United States Medical Licensing Exam), Step 1. Also, many medical schools will not award the coveted M.D. degree unless or until the student has successfully passed USMLE, Step 2, the clinical sciences portion of the national board examinations. It is not surprising, therefore, that so much planning, preparation, and emotion surround these tests.

But aren't medical students already very good test takers? After all, you took a lot of tests in your premedical years as college students and must have done well to be accepted to medical school. You probably survived intact the MCAT (Medical College Admission Test), VCAT (Veterinary College Admission Test), GRE (Graduate Record Exam), or whatever standardized test was required for admission to your school. What is so different now?

Medical School Tests Are Like Medical School Classes

The volume of information to be covered in medical school is much greater and more detailed than most students experienced in their previous education.

Much more detailed knowledge is needed on medical school tests than on previous tests. Few, if any, "general knowledge" questions appear on classroom or board examinations. Because every course must be passed, failure may mean dropping out or waiting a whole year to retake a class or return to school. Without question, testing creates a great deal of pressure. The importance of tests to medical students is reflected in the amount of anxiety associated with them.

A sound and systematic study plan is the best way to deal with pressure or fear of tests. If you have followed the SWS system thus far, you will be ready to "show your stuff" on the test. Knowing that you have covered the material as thoroughly as possible in the time between tests and that you have reviewed it regularly gives confidence that you will have the knowledge needed to answer most test questions. That detailed knowledge is acquired by systematic reading, note making, and review recommended in Chapters 3 and 4. You should have been over the information covered in the test at least five or six times before you take the exam (prereading, hearing a lecture, reading and note making, at least two reviews, and one self-testing session). In addition to mastering the information presented in the course, you will perform better on tests when you have reasonable insight into the expectations of your teachers and of the boards that govern licensure tests. The following will help you become "test wise," giving you a further edge when taking tests:

- Understanding test formats and efficient methods of approaching different types of test items
- Being alert to differences in instructions and to key words in each test item
- Preparing strategies to make the most of available knowledge
- Feeling physically and emotionally well during testing sessions

---

Learn to become test wise STAT!

Defining Terms

Before discussing good test-taking strategies, let's define the terms we will be using:

- The **stem** is the "question" part, or the stimulus to which the test taker must respond.

- **Response options** or **alternatives** are the possible answers on an objective test.
- Among these options, incorrect answers are called **distractors.**
- Among the options, correct answers are referred to as **keyed options.**
- **MCQ** is short for multiple-choice question.

Example

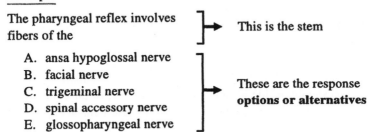

The pharyngeal reflex involves fibers of the → This is the stem

   A. ansa hypoglossal nerve
   B. facial nerve
   C. trigeminal nerve
   D. spinal accessory nerve
   E. glossopharyngeal nerve

→ These are the response **options or alternatives**

Answer

Response Option E is correct; thus, it is called the **keyed option.** It is the one listed in the key to the test. A, B, C, and D are called **distractors,** because they presumably distract you from the keyed option.

Commonly Used Types of Test Questions

Now that we are talking the same language concerning test items, let's look at the types of objective questions used in medical examinations. You should know all commonly used item types well and have their directions memorized in advance so that you don't have to take time to think about them during the test. In addition, strategies to optimize use of time or to make best use of available knowledge may differ among item types.

Because they are easily scored, often by optical scanning machines, most medical school tests consist of objective questions. These multiple-choice questions (MCQs) force you to think about relationships among pieces of information you have learned.

True-False Questions

True-false questions are not very common in medical education. But each option in the very popular multiple-choice question is a true-false question, so tips applying to true-false questions also apply to options in multiple-choice questions.

True-false questions usually relate two things according to a degree:

- All, most, some, none
- Always, usually, sometimes, never
- Good, bad
- Is, is not
- Positively related, not related, negatively related
- More, equal, less

Because each option in any multiple-choice item is actually a true-false question, you should decide whether any option is true or false, based on the information provided in the stem. For any true-false item, the possible responses are as follows:

   T = I know this is true
   F = I know this is false
  ?T = I think this is true, but I'm not sure
  ?F = I think this is false, but I'm not sure
   ? = No clue (This option was created by trolls in the dark of the
          moon for some course I have never taken.)

Tips for answering True-False Questions

After careful consideration, mark your decision in the margin next to the option according to the T, F, ?T, ?F, ? system. If any part of a true-false question is wrong, the whole question is false. Here is an example:

Example

True or False: *Axons* are *single fibers* that can vary in length from *less than an inch* to as *long as three feet.*

Explanation

This statement is true if, and only if, all four italicized sections are true.

Your basic strategy with true-false items is to read the stem very carefully and not miss any significant word in it. Because every part of the stem can be true except for one small word (e.g., *not*), you should underline any word or phrase that could make the question either true or false.

Unless incorrect answers are subtracted from total correct answers (penalty for guessing) always guess the answer—even when you haven't a clue about its correctness. Your odds with guessing are always 50:50 on true-false questions, which is a whole lot better than getting no credit for a blank.

One Best Response Multiple-Choice Questions

"One best response" is a multiple-choice question with a numbered stem and four or five lettered response options from which the test taker is asked to select the one **best** option. They are the most commonly used question types on board exams and are a mainstay of classroom exams. On boards, they are timed to take less than a minute each. Because most have five response options, you have only a few seconds to consider each option. You are usually allowed more time on classroom exams.

Always remember that you are looking for the **one best answer** when working with this item type. Other response options/distractors may be true but may not be as good as the best (keyed) option, as in the following example:

Example

Directions: Choose the best answer.

Scores on IQ tests are most highly correlated with which of the following?

F	A	Age
?F	B	Memory
?T	C	School achievement
?T	D	Socioeconomic status
F	E	Weight
F	F	Height

Explanation

Even with little knowledge of the subject you would quickly mark A, E, and F with an "F" for "false." But you may question options C and D, as shown with the "?T" marking. Go back to the stem and pay attention to the phrase "most highly correlated." It is probably true that socioeconomic class, school achievement, and IQ are all interrelated, but which would be "most highly correlated"? There is only one **best** answer.

When it is difficult to decide among possibly accurate responses, as indicated by your ?T notation, ask yourself a "why" question and mark a "because" reason briefly after the option. Returning the IQ item above, you would ask, "Why would school achievement be related to IQ?" Let's assume you know that schools often administer IQ tests to assess possible reasons for school failure, that parts of IQ tests are similar to school tests, and that it seems logical for school achievement to be related to intelligence. So you have three reasons to select C, even if you don't remember any specific bit of information from your lecture or text on this subject. Perhaps you can think of one reason for a relationship between social class and school achievement. You would make one- or two-word notes after each distractor to record your rationale. Because the preponderance of the evidence favors C, you would choose it, and you would be correct. Although socioeconomic status is to some extent related to IQ, the correlation between school achievement and IQ is higher. That is the one **best** answer.

The following example is of a *negatively worded* "one best response" MCQ.

Example

Which of the following substances is NOT secreted into the human digestive tract?

- F   A   Bile
- T   B   Insulin
- F   C   Trypsinogen
- F   D   Pepsinogen
- F   E   Ptyalin

Explanation

The *NOT* in the stem indicates that this item is **negatively worded**—that is, the *incorrect* answer is the keyed option. Insulin is the only alternative *not* secreted into the human digestive tract.

Negatively worded items can be confusing. Circle or underline the word in the stem indicating that the item is reversed or negative.

Four Tips for Answering One Best
Response Multiple-Choice Questions

1. Consider all the response options. As you do this, mark your decision on the margin next to the option according to the T, F, ?T, ?F, ? system. Wordy

items provide considerable information, which can give you hints, both in the stem and in the options. Although these more descriptive items can provide clues for answering with minimal or partial information, students often make careless errors by not paying attention to all the qualifiers in the stem or in various parts of the options. Here is an example from neuroanatomy.

Example

All of the following statements about a neuron that uses acetylcholine as its transmitter are true EXCEPT:

A. The key synthetic enzyme for the transmitter is acetylcholine transferase.

B. The synthetic enzyme for acetylcholine is found in the cytoplasm of the axon terminal.

C. The neuron relies on a powerful uptake mechanism to recapture acetate but makes choline intracellularly.

D. Acytelcholine is hydrolyzed by acetylcholinesterase.

E. The neuron could be a motoneuron or an autonomic preganglionic neuron.

It's easy to get lost in the wordiness of this kind of test question! Be careful not to make the following errors:

• *Forgetting that the stem is negatively worded.* This occurs when the options are so long and complicated that considerable time and focused attention goes to each one. After three or four such distractions, it's easy to forget part of the stem. You are looking for the exception here. All are true, EXCEPT . . .

• *Losing track of your decision about each option.* This happens for the same reason as number 1 above. For example, looking at the question above, you read Option A and think, "Hmmm, that sounds true." Then you read Option B and think, "This sounds right, but I'm not sure if it's only in the 'axon terminal.' " Reading C, you may think, "Probably not." You think D is true. You may then be uncertain about the E option; you know it could be a motoneuron but don't know if it could also be "an autonomic preganglionic neuron." Being so doubtful about E's accuracy, you select E as the one false answer, quite forgetting in the final emphasis on E that you also thought C was false or at least questionable. You will not make this mistake if you follow the recommendation to record your thoughts as T, F, ?T, ?F, or ? as you read each option.

• *Losing time because you did not leave a record of your thoughts as you read the stem and options the first time.* It is often the case that you need to return to an unanswered item. If you record the pattern of your original thoughts, you will save time as you reread all those lengthy options.

2. A word of admonition: Don't choose an alternative you've marked "?" over one you marked "?T." It seems incredible, but many test takers will select an option about which they know *absolutely nothing* over an option that they have some reason (partial knowledge) to think may be a good choice.

3. Eliminate all the options that you know cannot be correct. By this process of elimination, you can usually work the choice down to two options. For example, you may have worked your choice down to two options, one marked T and one marked ?T. Then you can examine every word in those two and select the one that is the best answer. If you have to guess, your odds of being correct are probably 50:50. If you have to guess, do not guess ?T over T. Never guess an option you marked as questionable (?), meaning that you have no reason to either choose or reject it, over one you marked as T or ?T, indicating that you had some reason to choose it.

4. On some test items, you should think of possibly making three different passes through a question:
   • Rapidly read it first and answer it immediately if you know certainly what should be keyed.
   • Second, if the first glance reveals a more difficult item, go back through the stem underlining key words, then systematically do the T, F, ? pattern for each option. Most students say this process works the choice down to two options that you can then examine more closely for key differences.
   • Finally, when all else fails, *guess*! If you've worked it down to two options, your odds of guessing correctly are probably 50:50.

A One Best Response Clinical Vignette

The clinical vignette is a special case of the one best answer MCQ, which are extremely popular on board exams. The questions consist of a description of a patient or problem situation and ask you to use your knowledge and apply it to this clinical situation. The stem may be very long and full of detailed information, possibly including patient history, signs and symptoms, laboratory findings, diagnosis, and/or treatment. This type of item is increasingly favored, because it points out the relevance and medical application of your basic scientific knowledge.

Example

A 48-year-old woman has had difficulty breathing, especially upon exertion, but also when resting. Blood pressure is 139/40 mm Hg; pulse is 79/min. Bilateral crackles are heard in both lungs, at the base. S_1 is normal, S_2 is diminished, and there is a short diastolic murmur along the upper left sternal border. The rest of the physical exam is within normal limits. An X-ray of the chest shows an enlarged heart. What is the most likely diagnosis?

    A. aortic insufficiency
    B. aortic stenosis
    C. mitral insufficiency
    D. mitral stenosis
    E. pulmonary insufficiency

Explanation

The strategic problem is mentally organizing so much information. If you were to underline key words, most of the stem would be underlined. In this case, a better strategy is to read the response options *first*. They are usually brief. After skimming through the possible answers, read the stem, searching for information that will relate to the response options and clues to help you rule each in or out and arrive at the correct one.

As a good test taker, you realize that these item types are too long to read repeatedly. You will need to answer each question to the best of your ability, without dwelling on it too long, and return to an item later if, and only if, you have new insight and the time to do so.

Matching

Matching questions are typically a series of items that test knowledge of closely related topics. These items consist of a lettered list of response options (usually five possible answers, lettered A, B, C, D, E) followed by a series of numbered questions or phrases, which are the stems. The task is to match each lettered option with its most-related word or phrase.

Example

Directions: The group of questions below consists of five lettered headings followed by a list of numbered phrases. For each numbered phrase, select the one lettered heading that is most closely related to it. Each lettered option may be used once, more than once, or not at all.

   A. Guaiac
   B. Bacitracin
   C. Cytochrome
   D. Nystatin
   E. Colchicine

   101. A fungicide
   102. An antibacterial cream
   103. A gout suppressor

Explanation

Matching questions are approached the same as one best response MCQ's. Read Number 101 and search Options A through E for the correct answer. Then go to Number 102 and so on. Matching items are also essentially a series of related true-false questions for which you ask yourself, "Option A is related to Number 101: true or false?"

Tips for Answering Matching Questions

Read the entire item (all numbered and lettered options in both columns) before making any choice. There may be some relationship between all possible choices in the item, but you are looking for the closest, or best, one.

Answer those you know first to get unknown relationships down to best odds on guessing.

You can also use the T, F, ?T,?F, ? strategy if you are having trouble with a matching item by making a small table in the margin. Write each lettered option as a column heading. Then ask about each possible response option, "Is this true, false, questionably true, questionably false, or no clue?" Mark your decision under the appropriate column heading. Using the items in the example above, your table might look like this:

A	B	C	D	E	
					101. A fungicide
					102. An antibacterial cream
					103. A gout suppressor

Matched Pairs

Another type of multiple-choice question is matching pairs, sometimes called "modified matching." The response options consist of two words or phrases (A and B), plus options to choose both or neither (C and D). Thus, you must know how both of the two main alternatives are related to the stem to choose the correct response. An example from behavioral sciences follows.

Example

Instructions: For each numbered word or phrase, select

A   if the item is associated with (A) *only,*
B   if the item is associated with (B) *only,*
C   if the item is associated with *both* (A) and (B),
D   if the item is associated with *neither* (A) nor (B).

A. Compulsive eating
B. Loss of appetite
C. Both
D. Neither

A	B		
?	?	11.	Anxiety
?	T	12.	Depression
T	F	13.	Bulimia
F	T	14.	Anorexia

Answer

Make a little table in the margin to record your true-false answers, as in the example above.

Tips for Answering Matching-Pairs Questions

The T, F, ? pattern on your little table gives you the keyed response, or if you have to guess, you can choose at least something that is questionably true rather than an option that is false or completely questionable. If you know one of the two matching pairs, you can reduce the odds of a wrong answer from 1:4 to 1:2.

Extended Matching

Increasingly popular on board examinations, extended matching items are essentially the same as regular matching questions, except there are more possible response options—as many as 26. Typically, the long list of options is paired with two to three questions.

Example

Directions: Choose the best answer from the list of options below.
Each answer may be used once, more than once or not at all.

A 35-year-old male reports he has been feeling tired and experiencing periodic chest pain for approximately four months. His other symptoms include a burning sensation in the chest and some nausea. These symptoms usually occur after meals. He is concerned because his father had a fatal heart attack at age 58.

The most critical possible diagnosis to investigate first would be:

A. Hypertension   G. Peptic ulcers
B. Cardiac insufficiency   H. Hypochondria
C. Mitral valve prolapse   I. Crohn's disease
D. Hypotension   J. Diabetes
E. Gastroesophogeal reflux disease K. Myocardial infarction
F. Spasm of the sciatic nerve   L. Hyperthyroidism

Tips for Answering Extended Matching Questions

Approach this item as if it were a short-answer question. You will not have time to carefully rule in and out each option. Read the test item, think of the answer, and find it in the list. Because "none of the above" is not an option, if you don't find the answer in the list of options, you'll need to return to the question. Repeatedly referring to the question can use up a lot of time, so mark any critical data the first time you read the stem.

There is less "cueing" on this item type than any other. You're not likely to simply recognize the correct answer, and the odds for guessing are not good. Still, a guess is always better than a blank, when there's no penalty for guessing.

Note that you are looking for "the most *critical*" possibility to rule in or out. It is possible that the most *likely* diagnosis is not the most dangerous health problem to rule out first.

Multiple-Multiple Choice

Multiple-multiple items are no longer used for national board examinations, but they may linger in classroom tests, as teachers are loathe to give up good items that took them a lot of effort to write. If these items do not appear on your class tests, you can skip this section. But if you anticipate having to answer multiple-multiples on midterms and finals, carefully study the patterns and strategies for answering, because, although they appear quite complicated on first acquaintance, their internal structure provides clues for correct answers or good guesses with partial knowledge.

Of four response options, the test taker must select one, two, three, or all four according to a fixed pattern.

Example

Directions: For the following question or incomplete statement, one or more of the answers or completions may be correct. Select:

A if only *1, 2, and 3* are correct
B if only *1 and 3* are correct
C if only *2 and 4* are correct
D if only *4* is correct
E if *all* are correct

1. This is a "multiple-multiple" choice item.
2. This is a "multiple-multiple" question.
3. You should pay particular attention to the pattern of true or false response options.
4. Guessing will be impossible.

When you see the directions above, you know

T 1. This is a "multiple-multiple" choice item.
T 2. This is a "multiple-multiple" question.
T 3. You should pay particular attention to the pattern of true or false response options.
?F 4. Guessing will be impossible.

<u>Explanation</u>

These directions do signal the (in)famous multiple-multiple choice, question. Using the T, F, ? system, you would choose "A" as the keyed option because 1, 2, and 3 are correct. We suspect D is false because of the specific determiner (or absolute) "impossible." It is possible to answer a multiple-multiple item correctly with only partial knowledge by carefully inspecting the true-false pattern, because only certain patterns are permitted. (See Figure 6.1 and the aid under "Tips for Answering Multiple-Multiple Questions").

Tips for Answering Multiple-Multiple Questions

Below is an aid for answering multiple-multiple questions:

IF	THEN
1 and 4 are both true	E is always the correct answer
3 and 4 are both true	E is always the correct answer
1 and 2 are both false	D is always the correct answer
2 and 3 are both false	D is always the correct answer
1 is false and 2 is true	C is always the correct answer
2 is true and 3 is false	C is always the correct answer
2 is false and 4 is true	D is always the correct answer
2 is true and 4 is false	A is always the correct answer

It is also possible to answer these questions more rapidly by making use of the pattern to eliminate the necessity of reading all response options. You could start with either Option (answer) 1 or 2, but just for illustrative purposes, in Figure 6.1, we show you how to "work" the pattern starting with Option (answer) 2.

General Test-Taking Strategies

Before the Test

Don't change your habits drastically just before a test. Make staying healthy a priority. Don't try a new diet. Avoid drugs of all kinds. Proctors tell horror stories about carrying sick students out of exams because they have overdosed on caffeine or over-the-counter pills to keep awake during the previous

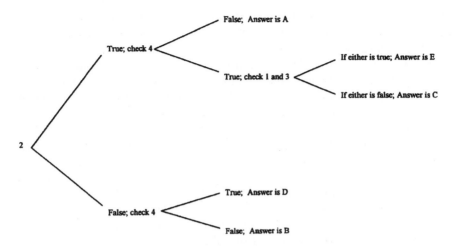

Figure 6.1. How to "Work" a Multiple-Multiple Choice Question

night(s). You want to be a health professional? Be sensible about your own health.

If you have incorporated the SWS system from the preceding chapters, it will be necessary to make only one additional final review of your condensed notes just before the test. Whether to self-test during this final review depends on how much anxiety doing so might create. If finding out what you don't know would reduce you to a quivering puddle, forget it. It wouldn't be worth it. If you tend to be more confident, self-test as you do your final review.

Remember, cramming does not pay! If you have reviewed the material regularly, it won't be necessary to stuff yourself with odd factoids at the last minute.

During the Test

Timing Considerations

1. First, quickly look over the test to decide how much time to spend per item and where you need to be on the test when half of the time has elapsed, then mark it on the test or answer sheet.
2. Next, answer the easy questions. This will aid in planning your use of time, and you will be sure to get credit for all the items you know. If you begin with the first test question and work straight through a test, you may run out of time before finishing and not receive credit for answers

you knew but didn't have time to answer. Answering the easy questions also builds confidence for your later attack on more difficult items.

3. If you get stuck on one question, make a note or mark in the margin and go on to other questions you can answer readily. You can come back later to the difficult ones. You'll find them quickly by the marginal note or mark. It sometimes occurs that the answer to an earlier item pops up at you in a later question about the same topic. In any case, if all the questions are worth the same number of points, it doesn't pay to sacrifice points on questions you can answer easily because you agonized too long over a difficult one.

4. Take the full time allowed for the test, even if you finish early. There is no advantage to leaving early. If you use the extra time to review the test, paying particular attention to items you noted with a question mark on the margin as uncertain, you may find errors, such as misreading part of the stem or option. If you discover that you made an error, you will have time to change your answer. (See below for tips on how to know when to change an answer.)

Example

Directions: Choose the one best answer.

You have two hours to complete a 60-item multiple-choice test. After working on the test for one hour, which item should you have reached?

    A.   Item #25
    B.   Item #30
    C.   Item #35
    D.   Item #50

Explanation

Did you answer 30, just because 30 is halfway through the test at half time? Actually, you should minimally be at **35,** because you probably did not finish each and every question and you'll need to return to those unanswered questions later. Good test takers make it a point to skim over the entire test before beginning to answer any question. They look for the total number of items and different types of items. They decide in advance where they want to be by the midpoint of the testing period. This assessment should include an estimate for time at the end to return to previously unanswered items.

Avoiding Careless Errors

Read the Instructions—and Believe Them! When the directions say "select the one best answer," you should:

    A.   Select what is most generally true
    B.   Choose an unusual exception (a "zebra")
    C.   Consider that none of the options may be a "best answer"

Clearly, you should follow the instructions and choose the best available option from among those offered, even if you could devise a better set of alternatives. Still, many students waste valuable test time arguing with the best available option, because they would have worded it differently or because they can recall some obscure exception to the general case. The first rule of test taking is *follow instructions*!

Marking the Answer Sheet. Have you ever arrived at the end of an answer sheet only to discover that you are marking the Number 99 space on the answer sheet for question Number 100? Sometime during the test, you skipped an answer blank. Horrors! You'll have to either erase the marks on the answer sheet back to the place where you got out of alignment, a terrible, time-wasting and anxiety-provoking task if your error was early in the test, or you will have to beg the teacher for mercy, if it's a classroom test.

If it is a standardized national exam, the scenario gets even worse. The strict time limits do not allow any extra time for correcting answer sheet errors. Your only hope is that, for an additional fee, you may request that the test be scored by a person, rather than a machine, so you can perhaps be given credit for correct answers even though you made a mistake in aligning your marks on the answer sheet. This nightmarish situation is easily preventable.

A simple way to avoid this problem: Check your marking alignment **every 10 items.** Every time an item number ends in zero, note that the answer sheet mark is on a line ending in zero. If you get off alignment, it will not take very long to correct the error.

When You Don't Have a Clue and Must Guess

1. If there is no penalty for guessing, do it. The directions for a test will tell you if points are subtracted for incorrect responses. In that case, you

probably shouldn't guess, although some test experts have argued that the odds of being ahead by guessing even then are fairly good. If you are running out of time, the best method, statistically speaking, for completing the answer sheet is to choose one letter and answer all the remaining questions with the same letter, straight down the page.

Example

Directions: For the following question or incomplete statement, one or more of the answers or completions are correct.

Regarding guessing:

A.   The good test taker will not leave any item blank if there is no penalty for guessing.
B.   You should not guess, because the test is supposed to measure what you actually know.
C.   You should choose the most unfamiliar option, because you may not have covered the material where it was mentioned.
D.   There is usually a penalty if you guess wrong.

Explanation

Option A.   True. Because this is one best answer multiple choice, you may stop here, although it would be prudent to skim the other options.

Option B.   The second part of the statement is true, but it does not follow that you should not answer each item if you want to maximize your score.

Option C.   Although students sometimes do this, it is not a good strategy for making the best guess.

Option D.   There is **not** usually a penalty for guessing. If there is, it should be clearly stated up front.

2. Stem-option repetition can be a clue to the correct answer.

Example

Directions: Select the one best answer.

All chordates are said to possess:

1.   a dorsal tubular nerve cord
2.   a vertebral column

3. jaws
4. appendages
5. a maxilla

Explanation

Let's suppose you have to guess on this one, and you've worked it down to a 50:50 choice between Options 1 and 2, because you know generally that chordates have some form of neural control system down the back. What you don't know is if they all have vertebrae. You can use the **stem-option** guessing technique here, if you must guess. A "stem-option repetition" means there is an exact repetition of one or more words, a repetition of part of a word, or a word in the option with the same meaning as a word in the stem. Here, part of the word *chordates* in the stem is repeated in Option 1 as *cord*, so that is the answer you would choose. Remember, you use this technique only *after* you have searched your knowledge base and looked at every part of the item and still can't choose better than a guess.

3. Specific determiners or absolutes can be a giveaway in guessing.

Example

Directions: Choose the one best answer.

All of the following are true regarding adenoviruses, EXCEPT:

A. The name derives from the fact that they were first found in children's adenoids.
B. Laryngitis is caused by an adenovirus.
C. Conjunctivitis, or "pink eye" is caused by an adenovirus.
D. They are a family of more than 40 viruses.
E. They never cause tumors.

Explanation

The giveaway in this example is the **specific determiner** *never*, even if you didn't know that adenoviruses can cause tumors in animals. *Always, never, inevitably,* and possibly *completely* are often clues to the incorrectness of a response option, because there is very little in life or nature that is so specifically determined. The option might be true if the adverb were *probably, sometimes, moderately, usually,* or *occasionally.*

4. Look for grammatical inconsistency between the stem and the option or other grammar cues.

Example

The internal intermuscular septum of the arm is perforated by an:

    A.   ulnar nerve
    B.   trigenimal nerve
    C.   optic nerve
    D.   condyle
    E.   deep fascia

Explanation

Because you know the answer is not any option that begins with a consonant (note the stem ends in *an*), you know it's between options A and C without any knowledge of the content! Grammatical inconsistency can also occur when the subject is plural in the stem and some response options are in the singular form (or vice versa). Because standardized tests are carefully tested before regular administration, grammatical cues will rarely occur in them.

5. Look for an absurd option. This may occasionally occur as a bit of levity offered by the teacher in a classroom test but is highly unlikely in a standardized examination.

Example

The origin of the epicranius muscle is the:

    A.   zygomatic bone
    B.   fascia in upper chest
    C.   occipital bone
    D.   funny bone

Explanation

You know that D is not the keyed option.

6. Look for a longer, more complicated or more complete option. In course examinations, you may be able to pick up a few points by becoming

familiar with the idiosyncratic test-writing style of a particular teacher. Some teachers tend to write keyed options that are longer than their distractors. These teachers want to add enough qualifiers to ensure a recognizable and defensible keyed option, readily distinguishable from the distractors. The extra qualifiers make the keyed option longer.

7. Look for a familiar option. If you must guess, choose an option that sounds familiar rather than one about which you know nothing or that you think you've never seen before. Oddly enough, some test takers select an option *because* they know nothing about it. Test questions are almost always based on information presented in the lecture, in the text, or in both. It is not a good idea to choose an option that is completely unfamiliar.

Example

The correlation between skateboarding and age is:

    a. positive
    b. negative
    c. nonparametric
    d. zero

Explanation

Obviously, skateboarding is a sport of relatively young people, so the answer is b. But some test takers who have no idea what the word *nonparametric* means would guess it anyway.

8. Look for similar options. Often, two options are alike except for one or two words, and the other options are all different.

Example

Directions: Choose the one best answer.

The structure running along the bicipital groove of the humerus is the:

    1. tendon of the long head of the biceps
    2. tendon of the long head of the triceps
    3. coronoid fossa
    4. styloid process
    5. ulnar artery

Explanation

Options 1 and 2 are the same except for the last word. If you know absolutely nothing about this topic, you will guess Option 1 because (a) it is one of a pair of similar options, which suggests that the test maker wanted to focus on the difference(s) between them, and (b) the repetition of the prefix *bi* in both stem and option (see stem-option guess above).

9. Look for a "good" or conscientious answer. When you haven't a clue, choose good things. A response option that seems more careful or conscientious (e.g., "It's important to obtain a thorough medical history when examining a new patient") should be considered "true."

Changing Answers

Students get conflicting advice about whether or not to change answers after they have recorded them on the answer sheet. Here's a question to help you untie this knotty problem.

Example

Regarding changing keyed options on previously completed items ("changing answers"),

   A. you should never change answers.
   B. research indicates that when students change answers, they always change from a correct response to an incorrect response.
   C. many psychiatrists say that changing answers is a sign of an obsessive-compulsive personality.
   D. you should change answers if you can think of a good reason to do so—for example, you now recall a fact that you didn't consider when originally answering the question.

Explanation

- Option A is probably wrong because it has a specific determiner: *never.* Options with specific determiners, such as *always, only,* or *never,* are usually incorrect.
- Research indicates that when students with higher grades change answers, they are more likely to improve their scores. These students probably changed their answers for a good reason, not just on a hunch. Again, the word *always* should have been a clue.

- Option C is an absurd choice, even if you haven't the foggiest notion what psychiatrists think about changing answers. Absurd, or jocular, options are usually distractors designed to give you a laugh and ease tension.
- Look at option D. This seems reasonable, doesn't it?
- The correct answer is D.

By the way, if you have a tendency to change answers on a hunch (no definite fact in mind), you should set up some barrier or reminder not to do it. Write something across the top of your answer sheet, such as "Never change an answer without a very specific reason." Carve a big question mark on your eraser to remind you to ask yourself, "Why am I erasing this? Do I have a good reason?"

Note on avoiding fatigue: If you feel tired when you are hungry, bring a snack to keep up your energy. Dried fruit and nuts are bite size and easy to eat. Don't bring anything big, messy, or noisy (either the food itself or the crackling of the wrapper.) Check with the teacher or proctor first, but most will allow you to bring something to eat if your doing so will not disturb others.

After the Test

It may not be very enjoyable to look at the mistakes you made on a returned test, but knowing why you missed a question can help keep you from making the same mistake again and is an important step to becoming a better test taker. We have some suggestions to help you develop a systematic technique for analyzing the errors you made each time you get back a scored test.

First, you need to identify the source(s) of your mistakes. Possible categories include the following:

- Insufficient information
- Failure to use good test-taking strategies
- Test anxiety
- Feeling physically unwell during the test

Count the number of items you missed that you can attribute to these four categories. Make a copy of and use the worksheet titled "Analysis of Test Errors" (Table 6.1) to identify the primary source(s) of the errors. See the example of the completed worksheet where there are two main sources of errors (Table 6.2). In this example, the student would have received an A on the test were it not for making six test-taking errors.

The student in the sample worksheet missed three questions due to lack of time for review. We would recommend that this student review the chapter on time monitoring and rework his or her study schedule to include enough time for review and self-testing. Almost all the test-taking errors could be eliminated next time. This student also needs to focus on timing issues related to testing. A review of this chapter just before the test might help him or her to avoid careless errors.

Don't give in to the temptation to slack off after an exam. It's OK if you sleep in for a couple of hours the day after a test, but after that, you should resume your regular schedule. Go back and skim Chapter 1 if you are tempted to take a big break right after a test. If you keep up your regular study habits, you'll be "cruising" while your classmates are cramming frantically before the next set of exams.

Exercise 1: Analyzing Test Errors

Go through a recently returned test and write the missed item number in the appropriate column on the "Analysis of Test Errors" worksheet. Answer these questions:

1. Was this information in the condensed notes (cards, charts, diagrams, etc.) that you used for review and self-testing?

   _____

2. If not, was that information presented in the lecture or required reading?

   _____

3. If it was presented only in lecture, did you miss that lecture?

   _____

4. If you did not get a good set of notes, was it because you did not preread before lecture?

   _____

5. Was the information missed a main idea or a detail?

   _____

Table 6.1 Worksheet: Analysis of Test Errors

Directions: Write the missed test item number in the appropriate column.

Insufficient Information	Did Not Use Good Test-Taking Skills	Test Anxiety	Physical/Health Problems	Description of Error
Totals				

Table 6.2   Sample Worksheet: Analysis of Test Errors

Directions: Write the missed test item number in the appropriate column.

Insufficient Information	Did Not Use Good Test-Taking Skills	Test Anxiety	Physical/Health Problems	Description of Error
15				Not in notes
	21			Left blank
33				Not in notes
		37		Couldn't think of answer
48				Didn't review
49				Didn't review
	54			Changed answer
	57			Didn't see "except" in stem
	72			Didn't see "not" in stem
88				From lecture, not in text
89				Didn't review
			96	Tired. Couldn't concentrate
	99			Out of time. Blank.
	100			Out of time. Blank.
Totals 6	6	1	1	

6. If it was a main idea, you must not have had it in your notes. If it was a detail, was it not attached somehow to its main idea?

_____

7. Sometimes the source of the error is such a "picky" detail that you wouldn't think of putting it in your notes. Chalk that error up to the test maker. Although, if there is a pattern of missing "picky" details, you may need to redefine *picky* and make more detailed notes!

8. If the information was in your notes, why didn't you remember it?

_____

9. Did you review it?

_____

10. How many times?

_____

11. Did you test yourself over it?

_____

12. How many times?

_____

Exercise 2: Doing Something About Test Errors

1. For the test results you analyzed in Exercise 1, what was/were your main source(s) of errors?

_____

2. How can you reduce this source of error on your next test?

_____

Students Say

"I'm a more efficient test taker. I have a system that I can use."

"Having a test-taking 'system' helps me stay calm during tests."

"I'm not making 'stupid' mistakes during the test!"

"The most helpful thing for me was learning to keep track of my responses using the ?, T, F system. I used to forget which answer I was leaning toward and would have to start over again!"

"I'm one of those who would get off track when marking the answer sheet. Now I check every 10 items and don't have to waste test time reentering my answers."

Summary

Test-taking strategies supplement the SWS system of mastering medical content. Being familiar with test formats and having strategies to avoid careless errors are no substitute for a solid knowledge of the material. You can, however, avoid losing points due to confusion over item construction, improper use of time, or failure to use all the information you possess. You will also approach tests with more confidence when you combine knowing the academic material thoroughly with being test wise.

If You Want to Know More

Bhardwaj, V. B., & Yen, E. Y. (1979). *Medical examinations: A preparation guide.* New York: ARCO.
   General advice and sample questions.

Biran, L. A. (1986). Hints for students (and examiners) on answering MCQ questions of the multiple true/false type. *Medical Teacher, 8,* 41-47.
   Discusses students' difficulties in tackling exam questions of the multiple true-false type.

Fabrey, L. J., & Case, S. M. (1985). Further support for changing multiple-choice answers. *Journal of Medical Education, 60,* 488-491.
   Review of research plus own study suggest the advice not to change answers is incorrect. Students who changed answers were twice as likely to improve test scores as to receive a worse score. Authors admit, however, that it is sound advice not to change an answer without a good reason.

Fleming, P. R., Sanderson, P. H., Stokes, J. F., and Walton, H. J. (1976). *Examinations in medicine.* New York: Longman.

   Reviews types of items that appear on standard medical examinations.

Frohlich, E. D. (Ed.). (1981). *Rypins' medical licensure examinations.* New York: J. B. Lippincott.

   Reviews types of items, gives test-taking advice, and offers many examples.

Hubbard, J. P. (1978). *Measuring medical education.* Philadelphia: Lea & Febinger.

   Overview of medical testing.

Jarecky, B. M. (1979). Preparing students for examinations. In W. E. Cadbury, C. M. Cadbury, A. C. Epps, & J. C. Pisano (Eds.), *Medical education: Responses to a challenge* (pp. 137-153). Mt. Kisco, NY: Futura.

   Describes test item types in tests taken by medical students and offers advice about test-taking skills.

Pappworth, M. H. (1985). *Passing medical examinations.* London: Butterworths.

   General information on test taking. Dislikes objective tests.

Sarnacki, R. E. (1981). *Test-taking skills: A programmed text for medicine and the health sciences.* Baltimore, MD: University Park Press.

   Very detailed review of item types and methods to make educated guesses when not sure of an answer.

Shahabudin, S. H. (1983). Patterns of answer changes to multiple-choice questions in physiology. *Medical Education, 17,* 316-318.

   Study of 4,000 Malaysian medical students tested the validity of the common advice that "first hunches are likely to be correct" and found that changing answers was more likely to correct an originally incorrect response than to alter an originally correct one.

7 Overcoming Test Anxiety

Diagnose Yourself: Physical Symptoms Scale

Just before or during an exam, some students report some of the following symptoms. Please indicate the extent to which each of the following affects you, according to the scale below.

0 = never/not at all   1 = rarely/slightly   2 = sometimes/a fair amount
3 = often/much   4 = very much/very often/always

Circle the appropriate number preceding each symptom.

0 1 2 3 4   1. Nausea
0 1 2 3 4   2. Constipation
0 1 2 3 4   3. Chills
0 1 2 3 4   4. Feeling dizzy/faint
0 1 2 3 4   5. Rapid heart rate
0 1 2 3 4   6. Muscular tension
0 1 2 3 4   7. Clammy hands
0 1 2 3 4   8. Headache
0 1 2 3 4   9. Dry mouth
0 1 2 3 4   10. Stomach cramps
0 1 2 3 4   11. Trembling
0 1 2 3 4   12. Diarrhea
0 1 2 3 4   13. Itching
0 1 2 3 4   14. Unsteady legs
0 1 2 3 4   15. Rash
0 1 2 3 4   16. Flushing

(0)1 2 3 4   17. Perspiration
(0)1 2 3 4   18. Chest pain
(0)1 2 3 4   19. Difficulty swallowing
(0)1 2 3 4   20. Ragged breathing

___8___   Total of circled numbers

Diagnose Yourself: Negative Thoughts

Just before or during an exam, some students report some of the following thoughts. Please indicate how often you might have the following thoughts prior to or during a test by circling the appropriate number, according to the scale below.

0. Never
1. Rarely
2. Sometimes
3. Often
4. Always

Preceding a test: (Questions 1-5)

0 1 2 3 (4)   1. I think, "I must get a good grade on the test or at least be above the class average."

0 (1) 2 3 4   2. I think, "If I get a low grade on the exam, I am stupid and worthless."

0 (1) 2 3 4   3. I think, "I'll never remember all this information; it's too much."

0 (1) 2 3 4   4. I think, "I'm going to fail."

(0) 1 2 3 4   5. I think, "If I fail this test, there'll be nothing to do with my life."

(7)

During a test: (Questions 6-12)

0 1 2 (3) 4   6. I think about how many questions I am not answering correctly.

0 1 (2) 3 4   7. I worry about how much time I have left.

0 1 (2) 3 4   8. I look around the room and think about how well others are doing.

0 (1) 2 3 4   9. I think "I can't answer this!" when I encounter a difficult item.

0 1 2 3 4   10. I sometimes think about things completely unrelated to the test questions.

0 1 2 3 4   11. I wonder what people, especially the faculty, will think of me when they see my test score.

0 1 2 3 4   12. I worry about my ability to pass the test.

_____ *12*   Total of circled numbers

☞ Stop.
Do not continue until you are ready
to score the Physical Symptoms Scale and
the Negative Thoughts Questionnaire

Scoring Directions: Physical Symptoms Scale

Add the total of the 20 numbers you circled.

Score Interpretation: Physical Symptoms Scale

If your total score is less than 10 (*and* you did not circle any 3s or 4s)—good news!—you do not appear to suffer from physical symptoms of test anxiety. You can skip this chapter.

If your score is in the 11 to 29 range, you could benefit from the information on relief of physical tension in this chapter.

If your score exceeds 30, or if you marked 3 or 4 in any two categories, you should read this chapter carefully and inquire about professional assistance in learning to relax in stressful situations. Your student counseling center may offer test anxiety desensitization training. It really works!

Scoring Directions: Negative Thoughts Questionnaire

Add the total of the numbers you circled.

Score Interpretation: Negative Thoughts Questionnaire

If you have 12 or fewer points—congratulations! You don't hurt your test taking and yourself with a lot with dysfunctional thoughts just before and during tests.

If you had 13 to 24 points, reading this chapter will save you some harrowing hours.

If you have more than 25 points, read this chapter carefully and perform all the suggested exercises. Some personal counseling might also help. Life can be better!

Anxiety

What Is Anxiety?

Fear is the appraisal of threat. Thus, if you are walking in the woods and see an irate bear charging toward you, it is perfectly normal, even wise, to appraise the situation as dangerous and to remove yourself as soon as it is safe to do so. Nature has evolved a complex system for warning us of imminent danger and preparing us to deal with it. When you see that bear in the woods, your eyes send a signal to the thalamus. The thalamus, in turn, relays the signal to both the amygdala and to the frontal cortex. The amygdala immediately triggers fear responses, including rapid heartbeat, perspiration, quickened respiration, muscular tension, and other physical responses that we call the "fight-or-flight syndrome." Unfortunately, we can neither run from nor fight most of the stressors in our modern environment. Medical school tests have little in common with bears other than being perceived as threatening.

We're also provided, however, with a mechanism for evaluating the nature of the threat. The thalamus sends a signal to the frontal cortex, which is slower to react than the amygdala. The signal from the thalamus to the frontal cortex is supposed to help you decide whether your perception of danger is accurate so that you can better control your physical response. In this chapter, it is our purpose to help your frontal cortex overcome the amygdala when you are preparing for a test and during a test. All that physical tension and unpleasant emotion just distract you from your task and impede your performance.

Relationship of Motivation to Anxiety

As motivation increases, so does fear or anxiety. If you perceive a situation as life threatening, your motivation will be extremely strong—and so will your physical and emotional responses.

You may ask, "But isn't motivation good for performance?" Yes, if it is kept at optimal levels. Psychologists describe the relationship between motivation and performance in terms of a curve (see Figure 7.1), which is found so consistently that it is called "The Yerkes-Dodson Law."

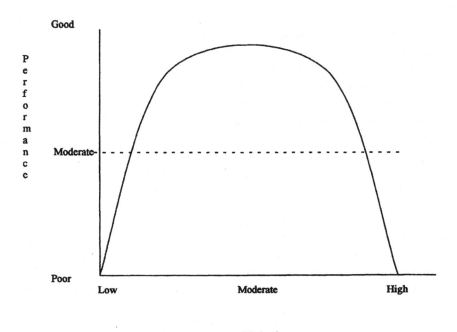

Figure 7.1. Motivation Versus Performance Curve

SOURCE: Yerkes, R. M. & Dodson, J. D. (1908). The relation of strength of stimulus to rapidity of habit formation. *Journal of Comparative Neurology, 18,* 458-482.

When motivation is low, so is performance. If you don't care much, you don't try very hard to succeed. When motivation is near the middle of that normal curve or average, performance peaks. When motivation becomes extremely strong, performance goes down. At the extreme, motivation becomes anxiety and its physical and emotional characteristics tend to interfere with performance. Scientific studies show that anxiety interferes with both learning (storage of information) and retrieval of information on tests. Test anxiety is motivation that is out of control.

Test Anxiety

To a highly motivated student, a test can be perceived as a threat. It is frightening to think of failing an exam. Fear causes the body to revert to its primitive amygdala-induced response. The heart beats rapidly to circulate more blood and oxygen to the brain and muscles. Muscles tense to strike or run. When the tension persists for a while, students can be subject to headaches, gastrointestinal disturbances, rashes, and other physical problems. If there were something physical to do with all that tension, it would be useful and good. But there isn't. You can't beat up a test. You just have to continue to sit there and try to focus your mind on making small marks on a piece of paper. The consequences of threat perception can be primarily psychological rather than physical—for example, constant worrying, self-doubt, not enjoying anything, or feeling chronically angry or irritable.

It has been estimated that as many as 15% to 20% of college students experience lower grades due to the effects of test anxiety. The actual percentage may be lower if we factor out tension or worry due to inadequate preparation. Test anxiety reduction programs do not usually deal with level of preparation or lack of knowledge of material to be covered on a test. Some very well-prepared students, however, have been known to suffer anxiety attacks during test administrations.

The most important difference between overanxious and not-anxious students is the difference in their ability to concentrate their attention on the test or pretest review. When taking an exam, the not-anxious student thinks only of whatever is necessary to complete the test as well as possible. Attention is fully focused on the test. The overanxious student may perform less well because attention is distracted by worrisome thoughts and/or physical tension.

If the diagnostic tests at the beginning of this chapter show that distracting and debilitating physical symptoms and/or dysfunctional thoughts just before and/or while taking tests are a problem for you, you will be glad to know that you can solve this problem in a relatively short time, if you are willing to work on it. Fortunately, much is known about how to keep your motivation in the right range—enough to keep you awake and alert, quick-thinking, and hardworking, but not so much that you have unpleasant symptoms and emotions. You *can* learn to control your anxiety.

Case Study

In anatomy class on Monday, the professor announces, "There will be a midterm this Friday on the structures of the head and neck." Student Doctor feels a distinct lurch somewhere in the vicinity of her stomach. She begins to wonder if she will be ready for the test by Friday. On Wednesday night, while reviewing her charts, diagrams, and cards on the structures of the head and neck, her heart starts beating faster as she worries about the possibility of not remembering the names and exact locations of all the structures. Her quickened heart rate indicates to her that there is a reason to be afraid ("My heart is pounding—there must be something to fear.") As she enters the classroom on Friday to take the test, she overhears some classmates quizzing each other about the facial muscles, and that starts her agonizing about whether she knows all of them. She begins to perspire. The answer to the first question on the test does not come to her immediately, and she thinks, "Oh, no, I'm going to fail!" Her heart is racing now. She looks longingly out the window and wishes she were anywhere else, but running away is no use and dreaming of elsewhere only wastes time, which is increasingly her concern. By the midpoint of the test, she has a headache from muscular tension in her neck and face, and her thoughts keep returning to how many questions she may have already missed. When she dots in her response to the last question on the answer sheet, there are five minutes left. She could go back and review some of those items where she made a best guess or was uncertain of the answer, but she just wants out of there. Student leaves early.

Student Doctor has not only violated some rules of good test taking, she has shown two kinds of anxious responses to the test-taking situation:

1. Physical symptoms of rapid heart rate, perspiration, muscular tension, and headache
2. Dysfunctional thoughts, including ruminating about what she does not know, imagining catastrophic outcomes, and dreaming of escape from the testing situation, culminating in leaving before the time she is required to hand in her test

Student was probably more aware of her physical symptoms than of her negative thoughts. Thoughts can proceed repetitively through the mind out of conscious awareness, a sort of background noise to which you don't pay attention. She could bring them to awareness with a little effort if she had a good reason to do so. If she did become more aware of her thinking patterns, she might notice that her negative thoughts (appraisal of threat) actually preceded her physical symptoms (flight-or-fight response) and reason correctly that she might be able to control her anxiety either by becoming more physically relaxed or by controlling her thoughts—or both.

Self-Control of Anxiety:
Two Basic Approaches

Just as there are basically two types of symptoms of anxiety (physical and cognitive), there are two fundamental approaches to the self-control of anxiety: physical relaxation and thought stopping (sometimes called cognitive behavior management, cognitive restructuring, or rational-emotive therapy).

Physical Relaxation

The physiological approach to anxiety reduction operates on the premise that it is not possible to feel emotionally anxious if you are physically relaxed. Various forms of relaxation training have been used in the treatment of test anxiety, including the following:

- Hypnosis
- Autogenic training (the repetition of certain words or phrases, such as "I feel calm," "My hands and feet are warm," etc.)
- Meditation (the repetition of one word or phrase slowly, while breathing deeply and rhythmically or focusing on a particular object and not permitting any thoughts to intrude on the blankness of your mind)
- Use of biofeedback equipment to decrease muscular tension or blood pressure
- Systematic desensitization

Instructions for all these methods are available on audiotapes, which may be available through your student counseling center or bookstore. Staff members at your counseling center may specialize in teaching students effective methods of relaxation. They also may offer individual or group test anxiety desensitization, a program that first teaches you self-control of relaxation, then moves you slowly and systematically from least anxiety-provoking simulated (imagined) testing situations to most threatening testing situations, while maintaining your relaxation response. Systematic desensitization has been documented for many years as an effective cure for test anxiety and can be taught to individuals or groups in a classlike setting.

It is quite easy to learn to relax your muscles systematically. This form of relaxation training is simply an organized version of what people do naturally when they stretch or yawn. If you suffer physical symptoms of anxiety, we suggest that you practice Exercise 1 next. Do the complete exercise at least once a day, preferably twice (once in the morning or early afternoon and once in the evening) a day, for the next few days. You will not only feel better and more relaxed, you will feel less tired. A 15- to 20-minute relaxation session has the effect of taking a nap.

Exercise 1: Systematic Muscular Relaxation

Instructions: Perform this exercise slowly and deliberately. It will take about 15 minutes. Pick a time and place to practice this relaxation exercise when and where you will not be disturbed or interrupted, preferably when you are alone in your own home. Take the telephone off the hook or turn off the ringer and the volume on the answering machine and turn off any other potential distractions, such as radio or television. Remove or loosen any tight clothing that would interfere with movement. Take off your shoes. Seat yourself in a comfortable chair that has arms and will support all the parts of your body when you let all your muscles go limp. Do not cross your legs. Put your feet flat on the floor in front of the chair. Sit with your spine rather straight against the back of the chair. Close your eyes so that you can focus on your internal sensations.

Do not worry whether you are successful in achieving relaxation. Just maintain a passive attitude and let relaxation come at its own pace. You will be systematically tensing and relaxing muscle systems, starting with your feet and moving up to your neck and head. It's a good idea to begin by noticing your breathing. Become aware of your breathing. Let your breathing become regular and rhythmic. Slowly fill your lungs and exhale. Each time you exhale, allow yourself to become more and more relaxed. If other thoughts intrude, just ignore them and gently let them go while you return to your practice of relaxation. When you feel that your mind is completely concentrated on your breathing and relaxation, let your thoughts turn to your feet.

You can begin by curling your toes toward the balls of your feet. Hold that position until you experience tension in the muscles of your feet and toes. Notice the tension. It is important to become very sensitive to the difference between tension and relaxation. Now, let all the tension go. Let all the tension flow away. Completely relax those muscles and notice the difference between tension and relaxation. Take a deep breath. Repeat this exercise. Enjoy how much more relaxed your feet now feel.

Now, turn your toes upward, as if you wanted to point them along your shins toward your knees. Stretch the muscles in that direction and pay attention to the tension that creates in your feet and along your shins. Hold the tension a while. Then let it go. Allow your feet to just relax. The tension seems to flow away. Enjoy the sensation of relaxation in your feet. Slowly take a deep breath. Then repeat the exercise to deepen the relaxation even more. Now point your toes downward so that they are in a direct line with your leg. Feel the muscles tense in your calves. Focus on that tension and hold it. And relax. Feel the tension go as a warm, comfortable sensation of relaxation flows into your feet and legs. Repeat this exercise to become even more deeply relaxed. Breathing slowly and deeply, let yourself sink deeper and deeper into a state of complete relaxation.

Now, tense all the muscles between your buttocks and knees. Hold this tension. Then relax and notice the difference. Repeat. Take a deep breath and relax. Arch your back forward and upward. Notice tension in the muscles down your back along the spinal cord. Hold that tension while you pay attention to how it feels. Then let it go all at once. Your back muscles now feel rather relaxed. If you would like to relax your back even more, arch your back again and let the tension develop thoroughly so that you will recognize back tension the next time it starts. Then let it all go and notice how your back feels when it is quite relaxed.

Let your thoughts now go to your shoulders. Hunch your shoulders together as if you were trying to make them meet across your chest. Hold that position and let the tension develop across your upper back. Release it all at once. Breathe deeply and enjoy the sensation of relaxation. Repeat this exercise to make your upper back completely relaxed. Now, pull your shoulders back, as if trying to touch them behind you. Hold this position long enough to let tension build up a while across your shoulder blades. Then release it all at once. Notice how good that relaxation feels. Repeat and focus your attention on the relief that comes with releasing tension in your back. Take a slow, deep breath as you relax even further.

You can relax the muscles of your neck. Let your head gently roll to the right until it almost touches your right shoulder. Feel the stretching along the left side of your neck. Hold it. Then release. Just let your head go back to its balanced upright position. Repeat until the left side of your neck feels completely relaxed. Then repeat this exercise to the left, stretching the muscles on the right side of your neck. Each time you release the tension of stretching, your neck feels more and more relaxed. Now let your head roll forward until your chin touches your upper chest. Feel the stretching in the back of your neck. Hold the tension for a while. Then let your head rise and relax. Slowly inhale and exhale and then repeat to more completely relax the muscles in the back of your neck. Now, push your head backward, stretching the muscles in the front of your neck. Hold the tension a while. Then release while breathing deeply and slowly. Your neck is feeling very relaxed now, but you can relax even more by repeating the stretch on the front of your neck.

After you have savored the sense of relaxation in your neck for a while, allow your thoughts to move to your jaw. Clench your teeth and feel the muscles of your jaw and temples tighten. Pay attention to this tension so that you will recognize it when it occurs at other times. Then relax. Let all the tension go. Take a deep breath and move your jaw around to loosen the muscles and be sure they are completely relaxed. Let your jaw go slack. Let your mouth hang open for a while. Take a deep breath and enjoy the feelings of relaxation that are progressing all over your body. It is very pleasant to just let your muscles go loose and feel completely relaxed. You can relax the many muscles of your face by squeezing your eyes tightly shut, pushing your eyebrows together across your nose, and pursing your lips into a tight little circle. This is not an exercise you want to do in a public place, but go ahead and let your facial muscles all become very tight in this way, since you are alone. Hold the tension as long as you can and then let go. Breathe deeply and slowly. Relaxation feels so good after tension. Repeat until your face feels smooth and relaxed.

Now you are feeling relaxed all over your body. You can continue to passively enjoy sinking into a deeper and deeper state of relaxation with each breath. When you inhale, let your chest expand fully and you fill your lungs. When you exhale, let your whole body go limp and relaxed.

When you want to arise and become active again, do so slowly. Begin by wiggling your fingers and toes. Then open your eyes and survey your surroundings. You may want to just sit there for a while with your eyes open. When you are ready, stretch and yawn. Take time to move as you would when arising from a night of slumber. You will feel rested, relaxed, and ready for the activities of your busy day.

If you find it difficult to perform this exercise from written directions, record these exercises yourself or buy or borrow an instructional audiotape. Prepare your room and yourself for a relaxation session before turning the tape on. Remember that your practice should occur well in advance (two to four weeks) of its need in a stressful situation where the skill will be used.

Many people become so proficient at self-controlled relaxation that they do not require any analgesic for minor dental or medical procedures.

Exercise 2: Reflections and Feedback
on the Systematic Relaxation Exercise

Fill in the blank.

1. Immediately after my relaxation exercise, I feel

   _____

2. When I have become physically relaxed by my 15-minute exercise, I notice that I stay relaxed for about _____ minutes or _____ hours afterward.

Practice makes perfect. When you have become skilled at controlling muscular tension and feeling relaxed, move on to the following exercise. Exercise 3 should be completed only after successfully practicing the relaxation exercise at least three times, to ensure proficiency.

Exercise 3: Systematic Desensitization

Do this exercise at least one week before an exam. Take 15 minutes to become thoroughly relaxed using the instructions in Exercise 1. When you feel deeply relaxed, imagine that you are actually taking the test that is coming up next week. See yourself sitting in the testing room. Imagine the other students sitting there, too. Imagine the chair you will be sitting in while you take the test. Try to sense how the chair feels as it touches your body. Imagine the teacher or proctor distributing the test and giving instructions. In your mind's eye, see the test paper on the tabletop or desk in front of you. Try to make this as realistic as possible. Then allow yourself to feel some slight tension or anxiety as you visualize the test-taking situation. As soon as you feel the sensation of tension or anxiety, repeat the relaxation exercise (#1) above until the tension completely disappears and you once again feel relaxed, calm, and comfortable. If you are able to successfully eliminate all tension produced by your visualization of the test setting with this relaxation exercise, then keep repeating it daily until the date of the exam.

The purpose of this exercise is to provide practice to proficiency in achieving voluntary relaxation, even in the face of a normally tension-producing situation. If you are unable to eliminate physical tension during this exercise, do not continue on your own. Seek professional help to desensitize your test anxiety.

A word of warning: Students enrolled in anatomy have reported that systematically relaxing different muscle groups sometimes leads their thoughts toward their anatomy course and interferes with relaxation. If you start to obsess about the name, function, or point of insertion of the muscles as you do this exercise, we recommend you try autogenic training or one of the meditative approaches to physical relaxation, although they tend to be harder to learn without the aid of a teacher or audiotape.

Exercise 4: Meditation Exercise

Learning to meditate on your own is paradoxically very simple and very difficult: simple because the instructions are minimal and the task (clearing the mind) seems uncomplicated; difficult because it requires passive concentration or attention, not typically a highly developed skill for most people in our fast-paced world. Give it a try. . . .

To begin, find a quiet place. Sit in any comfortable position with your back straight (against the chair back, if in a chair). Close your eyes, bring your full attention to the movement of your breath as it enters and exits your nose. Focus on the flow in and out of the nostrils. Don't follow it into your lungs or out into the air. Note the full passage of each in-and-out breath. Each time your mind wanders to other thoughts or is distracted by background noises, gently bring your attention back to the easy, natural rhythm of your breathing. Just be aware of your breath. Don't try to control it. Whether your breathing is fast or slow, deep or shallow, it is your attention to it that matters. If you have trouble keeping your mind on your breath, count each cycle of inhalation and exhalation up to 10, then start over again. The counting doesn't matter, just your attention. Meditate like this for 20 minutes. You can set a timer or peek at your watch when you think 20 minutes have passed. For best results, meditate twice a day in the same place and at the same times.

This is a simple exercise, requires no equipment, and can be performed away from home. Forms of meditation have been used almost everywhere in the world for calming the mind, focusing attention, or religious purposes. Instruction may be available in your community. Audiotaped instructions are also available, but as you can see, it is less a matter of guidance, than of passive concentration. Those who meditate regularly report that a 20-minute session has the effect of a refreshing nap.

Self-Control of Worrisome Thoughts

Systematic programs have also been developed to gain control over unnecessarily negative perceptions of life situations. This section discusses the second primary method of controlling test anxiety.

Proponents of thought stopping would argue that it is precisely the frightening appraisals (negative thoughts) about a situation that cause the physical symptoms (bodily preparation to deal with the threat) in first place. You have to see, or think you see, an angry bear before a signal goes to your nervous system to start the fight-or-flight response. If you don't see a bear or if you perceive the bear as Winnie-the-Pooh, then you don't become alarmed. Thus, it is more efficient to prevent physical symptoms by stopping negative thoughts as soon as they occur. The trick here is to identify those thoughts instantly (before they have a chance to get your body alerted) and to develop fast and effective ways of replacing them with more positive, or at least more functional, thoughts.

Patterns of Negative Thinking

Negative thoughts tend to fall into six main categories:

1. I'm awful. I'm not the kind of person who succeeds. I'm just not good enough. It's all my fault.
2. You're/they're awful. You/they are wrong to do this to me. You/they are harming me. It's all your/their fault.
3. I can't. There is nothing I can do about the situation. I am caught hopelessly, helplessly in this dilemma, problem, or situation.
4. This is killing me. What is happening to me right now is unbearable.
5. Fantasy. I should have a genie in a bottle or a helpful fairy godmother. Things should be better and easier. My life shouldn't be hard. I shouldn't have to work for things; they should just come to me.
6. Doomsday. My future is bleak. Something terrible is going to happen—sooner or later. I will soon be destroyed by whatever is tormenting me.

Any of the six main categories of negative thinking can adversely affect studying and test taking.

- It's hard to concentrate on your text or notes when you are covertly saying to yourself, "Forget it. You're a loser."
- It's also hard to keep positively focused on your academic task when you think your teachers are out to get you: "They plan to fail half the class."
- The "I can'ts" make you give up too soon when persistence is required: "I need a break. I can't concentrate more than an hour at a time. I can't sit here and look at these test questions one more minute!"

- Making a monster of the academic task ("It's driving me crazy!") could lead to avoiding necessary work.
- Fantasizing about how much better life should be might lead to stopping work early and heading for the basketball court or a party, because you think you deserve a good time or at least a break. The test taker whose eyes wander to the clouds floating by out the classroom window, dreaming of hiking through a gorgeous mountain meadow, has escaped via fantasy.
- But perhaps the worst pattern for test takers is inevitable impending doom: "I will answer this question incorrectly. Then I will fail this test. Then I will fail this course. Then I will flunk out of medical school. Then my life will be ruined." Some people have this pattern so well established that they can go directly from "I don't immediately know the answer to this question" to "My life is over" in two seconds flat, without bothering with any intermediary doomsday thoughts!

People tend to have favorites among these patterns of negative thinking. A world-class negative thinker can use all six patterns! For the most part, these thoughts just flow unheeded like the background noise of traffic on a busy street, but perhaps you can already identify the one(s) you prefer when you feel threatened.

If you suffer from negative thinking, work through all the following exercises until you are thoroughly familiar with this four-step concept. The first three steps are as follows:

- Step 1: Identifying the situation in which the problem occurs
- Step 2: Discovering the underlying thought
- Step 3: Realizing the consequence, or what happens (behavioral or emotional response) as a result of your negative self-talk or thought

Exercise 5: What's the Underlying Thought?

The situation or activating event (1) is supplied, as is the behavioral or emotional response (3), but the negative thoughts (2), are not present. You are to determine what thought might have been there to connect the situation (1) with the emotion or behavior (3). Write in the thought that would logically account for each sequence.

1. Student is at the first station of a gross anatomy practical exam. Student has test blank and pencil in hand and looks at the first exhibit.
2. The student thinks _____.
3. The student screams and runs out of the room.

1. Student is seated in study area at home making a final review of the material before a major test.
2. Student thinks _____.
3. Student puts head down on the desk and weeps.

1. Student is in the middle of a final examination.
2. Student thinks _____.
3. Student's shirt is dripping wet from perspiration and his hands are trembling as he fills in responses on the answer form.

1. Student, during a board exam, keeps looking around the room at other test takers.
2. Student thinks _____.
3. Student feels tense and anxious.

Exercise 6: Discovering Your Patterns of Negative Thought

Keep a little notebook in your pocket for a week. Every time you become aware of negative, unproductive self-talk, jot the thought in your notebook. This will help you identify your own pattern of negative thinking.

What did you learn from this exercise?

_____

_____

Exercise 7: Analyzing Thoughts Using the Four-Step Method

Now that you are familiar with the 1, 2, 3 sequence, tear out the worksheet in Table 7.1 and make additional copies if you want more practice on analyzing your thoughts. Using two different worksheets, describe what you thought in two different situations (1s) and how your thoughts (2s) led to specific outcomes (3s) for you. Most people notice only the first and third factors and are unaware of the underlying thought. Those who learn to identify the thought, however, are on the way to changing the outcome.

Table 7.1   Worksheet: Analyzing Your Thoughts Using the First Three Steps of the Four-Step Method

1. Describe the unpleasant situation, unfortunate circumstance, your own behavior, another person's behavior, or whatever experience preceded your feeling.

_____

_____

_____

_____

_____

_____

2. Thoughts about the situation: Describe what you thought about the situation and what you said to yourself about the event.

_____

_____

_____

_____

_____

_____

3. Consequences of your negative thought: How did you feel and behave as a result of your thoughts?

_____

_____

_____

_____

_____

_____

Why Change the Way You Think About Studying or Taking Tests?

When students allow themselves to fall into negative thinking patterns, they report feeling frustrated, worried, depressed, sad, anxious, afraid, angry, panicky, hurt, discouraged, defeated, and tired. Were any of these unpleasant emotions a consequence for you in Exercises 6 or 7 above? Wouldn't you like to replace those negative thoughts with more accurate and realistic assessments of the situation, to feel more calm, confident, motivated, energetic, enthusiastic, relaxed, hopeful, and ready to "hit the books" or "dive into" the test question?

You *can* learn to change the way you think about things. Learning how to change thoughts and feelings involves more than just saying "no" or "stop that." You will probably have to take some time to go through a process in which you force yourself to be more aware of those intermediary thoughts, question their validity, and develop more useful replacements. Specialists who teach people how to gain self-control over their thoughts and feelings have found that it helps to go through a complete four-step analysis whenever negative thinking is a problem.

The first three steps are the now-familiar situation (1), underlying thought (2), and emotional or behavioral response (3). The fourth step is challenging the thought that causes problems. You challenge it by asking three questions:

1. Is it **true**? Most of the time, the answer is no, and you can decide to reject the thought without further ado. Most anxiety-producing thoughts are exaggerations of possibilities and are not exactly true.

2. Even if the thought is true, or partly true, is it **useful** to think it at this time? Usually, the answer again is no. For example, maybe the test question is very difficult (there are usually at least a few difficult questions on most tests). How does it help you to spend time and get tense about that fact when you really should be putting your time and mental energy into figuring out how to deal with the question?

3. Finally, does thinking this way help you **achieve your goals**? The answer again is usually "no," if the consequences are painful feelings that interfere with studying and concentrating on tests. If your immediate goal is to concentrate your attention entirely on the TCA cycle (or whatever the topic of that difficult question), then this belief is certainly interfering with that goal. Put all your thoughts and energy in the direction you want to go.

4. After asking yourself those three questions, there is one further consideration: Do you want to reject this negative thought?

If the process of challenging these negative thoughts convinces you to reject them, you will then need to replace them with a more accurate or more useful thought that is consistent with your goals. Be very careful that your replacement thought is both true and believable, or your mind won't buy it. For example, if you generally receive an average grade on tests, it would probably be neither true nor believable for you to replace the failure self-talk with the thought that you will ace the test. It's too big a stretch from "I'm going to fail this test," to "I'm going to get 100% correct." But it would probably make sense to think, "I'm going to pass." And remember, "P = M.D.!"

Do not use any negative word in your new replacement thought. For example, you would not think, "I won't fail." The very word *fail* is too threatening, and you might not succeed in altering your unwanted physical or emotional response. Some generally true, believable, and positively stated replacement thoughts might be the following:

"I am carefully following a good study plan that will help me on the test." This is at least a neutral statement. Neutral is better than negative.

"I may not get the top grade on this test, but I will certainly pass it." This goes beyond neutral to anticipating a positive outcome—passing.

"Thousands of medical students have passed this course. If thousands pass each year, the odds are that I will, too." Again, positive.

"I really enjoy this course. The more I enjoy it, the more I want to study." This is a winning combination. This replacement thought goes beyond just acceptance to welcoming the challenge.

Beginners in disputing and replacing negative thoughts may want to aim at first for at least a neutral new thought. Welcoming all of life's tough challenges might be saved until at least a steady neutral state has been achieved. Always frame your replacement thought so that it points you in the direction you want to go. For example, "I am becoming better and better at taking tests." You might as well point yourself in that direction, as you have many more ahead of you!

Exercise 8: Changing Your Thoughts

This exercise asks you to perform a complete 1, 2, 3, 4 analysis (see Table 7.2). In this exercise, you will practice disputing the negative thought and decide whether you want to change it. If you decide that a replacement thought will cause a better consequence or outcome for you, you are asked to develop your own new replacement thought. Tear out the worksheet in Table 7.2, make additional copies, and carry one with you to analyze a negative thought when one occurs.

Practice Makes Perfect (Or at Least Good Enough)

Thinking is just covert behavior and can be changed like any other behavior that causes problems. Changing habits requires attention and practice. If you have for many years established a habit of using certain patterns of unproductive, negative self-talk, you will need lots of practice in catching your old dysfunctional thoughts and changing them quickly before they cause problems. Table 7.3 reviews six types of dysfunctional thinking and helps you figure out how to deal with them. You want to develop a new habit of sensible thinking well in advance of a situation in which you will need to use it effectively.

Exercise 9: Practice Thought Stopping

Two or three weeks before a test will probably be a good time to complete this exercise. Allow yourself about 10 minutes each time you repeat it. Do it once a day or every time you notice that you are having a problematic thought. If this much repetition becomes boring, all the better! Boredom is rarely associated with anxiety. By the test date, you should have talked yourself out of your dysfunctional thinking.

1. First, say out loud (or write on a piece of paper) the thought that bothers you. You need to get it out in the open. For example, you could say, "I am going to fail the biochemistry test in three weeks." You have explicitly identified your belief as probable failure.

2. Second, ask yourself what is the consequence of thinking you will fail this test in three weeks. Some logical consequences might be that you would feel tense, nervous, irritable, depressed, and possibly have any

number of unpleasant physical symptoms after experiencing this tension for a while.

3. Now, ask yourself, "Is my belief that I will fail true? What facts do I have to prove that I will definitely fail? What are the real odds that I will be one of the few people who will fail the test, especially given that I have faithfully adopted the SWS study system? Is the belief an exaggeration?"

4. Finally, ask yourself, "If there is even a grain of truth in my belief that I will fail the biochemistry test, what good would it do me to continually think it?" Look back at your responses to the diagnostic tests at the beginning of this chapter. Do you really **want** to continue to have these symptoms of test anxiety? The answer has to be a resounding NO!

5. Decide to replace the dysfunctional thought with one that is true, believable, and does not cause you problems. Be certain that your replacement thought is stated in positive, or at least emotionally neutral, terms.

6. Say your replacement thought to yourself until you believe it. Concentrate and focus your attention on the replacement thought until it really has erased the original dysfunctional one.

You should practice this exercise on a daily basis until you have erased your former thinking habit. You can copy and complete the 1, 2, 3, 4 worksheet in this chapter, if that would help you go through the process. You can also carry a practice 1, 2, 3, 4 form with you as you go to your classes and labs so that you will be prepared to deal immediately with any negative self-talk as it occurs. As you become proficient with practice, the process will come more naturally, and you won't have to go through each step. You will go directly to more sensible self-talk. And you will feel much better.

Exercise 10: Using Physical Symptoms to Identify Negative Thoughts

Every time you feel a physical symptom of tension, for example, your stomach seems to turn over or squeeze, immediately look for the preceding thought. Then do a complete thought-changing exercise (1, 2, 3, 4) to get rid of it and replace it with one that is true, believable, and does not cause problems.

Exercise 11: Combining Thought Changing With Relaxation

If you suffer from both the physical and emotional symptoms of test anxiety, you can actually work on eliminating both at the same time. Go back to Exercise

Table 7.2 Worksheet: Analyzing Your Thoughts Using the 1, 2, 3, 4 Method

1. Describe the unpleasant situation, unfortunate circumstance, your own behavior, another person's behavior, or whatever experience preceded your feeling.

_____

_____

_____

_____

2. Thoughts about the situation. Describe what you thought about the situation and what you said to yourself about the event.

_____

_____

_____

_____

3. Consequences of your negative thought. How did you feel and behave as a result of 1 and 2?

_____

_____

_____

_____

Given the consequences, do you wish to retain Number 2?   _____ Yes _____ No

If your answer is no

4. Challenge the thought. Argue with yourself by asking these questions:

   a. Is this thought *true*?

   b. Even if true or partly true, is it *useful* to think this at this time?

   c. Does thinking this help me *accomplish my goals?*

If you decide to discard your negative thought, write your replacement thought below. It should be accurate, believable and lead to more positive or at least more calm, feelings.

_____

_____

Table 7.3 Summary of Six Types of Dysfunctional Thinking, Consequences, and Replacements

Type of Thought Pattern	Unproductive Self-Talk	Consequence	More Useful Replacement Thought
I'm awful	If I get a low grade on the exam, I am stupid and worthless.	Depressed. Want to give up. Feel tired. Lose motivation.	If I make mistakes, I'll learn from them and do better next time. I have many good qualities, and will use them to perform at my best level. Maybe even Einstein didn't always get good grades. I'll just do my best!
They're awful	The teacher will flunk half of the class!	Angry. Complain.	What are the odds that half of the class would flunk? This teacher expects a lot, but I will try to meet her expectations. Realistically, they probably aren't even thinking about me. I am not the target.
I can't	I'll never learn all this information; it's too much.	Don't persist. Feel anxious. Helpless.	One step at a time. First I'll organize this material into related segments and make notes of the most important facts.
It's killing me!	I can't sit here one more minute. I've got to get out of here!	Terrified. Fear. Avoid the task at hand.	Take a deep breath and relax. Sitting here another 10 minutes is not that hard. Focus on the next step. Look for the next easy thing to do—to get back into it.
Fantasy	This should be easier. I shouldn't have to work so hard.	Waste time. Daydream. Lose concentration.	Things don't have to be easier. Who ever said medical school would be a "rose garden"? It's not easy, but it can be done.
Doomsday	If I fail this test, there'll be nothing to do with my life.	Dread. Fear. Worry. Distraction.	All I need to do is stick my nose back in my work. I want to concentrate my attention on the subject at hand.

1 and use this method to become very relaxed. When you are deeply relaxed, allow yourself to think just briefly the undesirable thought, "I'll fail," for example. You will probably experience some tension as soon as you have this thought. Tense and relax your muscles again and concentrate on the replacement thought you selected earlier. Say it to yourself with strong emphasis. Say it repeatedly. Then relax again. The purpose of this exercise is to expunge negative thinking and develop the habit of useful self-talk in a pleasantly relaxing atmosphere.

We hope the exercises in this chapter help you keep your motivation in the optimal range as you take tests. You want to be physically relaxed and mentally alert, with your thoughts tightly focused on answering the questions with maximal skill. If you need additional help in dealing with either tension or worrisome thoughts, we urge you to talk to a professional counselor at your student counseling center. You might benefit from more intense work with the methods outlined in this chapter, or you may find that other methods—for example, hypnotism, biofeedback training, or one of the types of meditation— would work well for you. All have proven successful in relieving test anxiety.

Students Say

The following quotations are taken from students who practiced replacing negative thoughts.

I used to think, "I'm failing this anatomy test!" I then felt scared, helpless, and depressed. Now I think, "I'll do my best." I feel I'm coping well.

I used to think, "I'm dumb, slow and mentally handicapped." When I thought that I felt dumb, slow, mentally handicapped and all-'round rotten and tired." Now I think, "I'm improving on each test slowly but surely, and I'm getting better." I now feel more confident, more motivated, and able to concentrate better.

I used to think, "I can't remember all this information!" That made me feel anxious. Now I think, "Stop! Break it up into small chunks. You can remember small parts." When I substitute this kind of thought, I feel hopeful.

When I sat down to take a test, I often thought, "I'd rather be anywhere but here." I let my mind wander. Now I say to myself, "This information is really interesting. It will be very useful to me." I can concentrate better now.

I used to think, "I have the worst brain of anyone in my class! There's no way I can remember this material well enough to be a good doctor." That made me feel anxious. Now I make it a point to say to myself, "This material is fascinating. I'm going to jump in and do as much of it as I possibly can." Now I feel enthusiastic and more positive about my classes in general.

I said to myself, "My grade on this biochemistry test is terrible, and I'm not a very good student." That made me feel uptight, frustrated, and depressed about my capabilities. Now I keep saying to myself, "I'm going to work very hard and do my best to improve my grade." I feel much better and ready to hit the books and work hard to learn.

I kept telling myself, "Face it, you're no good at taking tests." That made me feel sad, afraid, and inferior. Now I work at saying to myself, "I am good and smart enough, and I will do the best I can." I feel more confident and happy. It turns out my stress was a much larger factor in my performance than were my study habits!

I thought, "I'll never pass this test. There's too much information." That made me panicked and afraid. Now I concentrate on saying to myself, "Everyone has the same amount of time. There is enough time to get through the information—especially if I'm organized." What I needed most to improve my grades was to confront my attitude problem. It was only after facing the fact that I was doing it to myself and battling with myself for a more positive attitude that I began to improve.

I used to wonder, "How am I ever going to get through all this material?" (implying, "I'll never get through"). Then I felt depressed and tired. Now I make myself think, "I have a good system of studying, and it is working." I feel more confident and am also spending more time studying and enjoying it more.

Summary

For most medical students, the SWS approach to learning will by itself eliminate disabling test anxiety. When you have mastered the medical content, you may even look forward to the opportunity to use your knowledge on a test.

For an additional percentage of students, having well-established good test-taking strategies lends confidence: You know what to do at any given time during a test.

A relatively small percentage of students continue to experience distracting symptoms of test anxiety, even when they are test wise and well-prepared academically. We hope that understanding the biological basis of your symptoms and practicing one or both of the two basic approaches to getting rid of them has been helpful to you. We wish you well as you move forward to meet the challenges ahead.

If You Want to Know More

Benson, H. R. (1976). *The relaxation response.* New York: Avon.

A physician's guide to a simple meditative method of relaxation that proved effective with heart patients.

Deffenbacker, J. L. (1980). Worry and emotionality in test anxiety. In I. G. Sarason (Ed.), *Test anxiety theory, research and applications.* Hillsdale, NJ: Lawrence Erlbaum.

Reviews research on the importance of worry in test anxiety and discusses implications for treatment.

Denny, D. R., & Rupert, P. A. (1977). Desensitization and self-control in the treatment of test anxiety. *Journal of Counseling Psychology, 24,* 272-280.

Both desensitization and self-control are effective in reducing debilitating test anxiety, but teaching students how to cope with physical tension is more effective in improving test performance.

dePablo, J. S., Subira, S. Martin, M., deFlores, T., & Valdes, M. (1990). Examination-associated anxiety in students of medicine. *Academic Medicine, 65,* 706-707.

Medical students had increased anxiety depending on the importance attributed to the test, but not to its difficulty.

Ellis, A. (1971). *Growth through reason.* Palo Alto, CA: Science & Behavior Books.

Ellis is the originator of thought stopping as a way to improve emotional well-being. He writes in a nontechnical readable style with considerable humor. Not specifically about test anxiety, but his book is useful for the general purpose of keeping your feelings under control.

Ellis, A., & Harper, R. (1971). *A guide to rational living.* North Hollywood, CA: Wilshire.

See note above. Ellis's books are generally available in libraries and bookstores.

Finger, R., & Galassi, J. P. (1977). Effects of modifying cognitive vs. emotionality responses in the treatment of test anxiety. *Journal of Consulting and Clinical Psychology, 45,* 280-287.

Controlling thoughts alone is as effective in reducing test anxiety as relaxation training or a combination of relaxation training with thought control.

Goldfried, M. R., Linehan, M. M., & Smith, J. L. (1978). Reduction of test anxiety through cognitive restructuring. *Journal of Consulting and Clinical Psychology, 46,* 32-39.

College students who participated in systematic rational restructuring groups had significant decreases in subjective anxiety during test taking.

Greenberg, D. (1966). *How to make yourself miserable (a vital training manual).* New York: Random House.

A humorous approach to worry, with many funny cartoons to illustrate that you can ruin any situation if you are an outstandingly negative thinker.

Hembrie, R. (1988). Correlates, causes, effects, and treatment of test anxiety. *Review of Educational Research, 58,* 47-77.

Reviews 562 studies of test anxiety and concludes that test anxiety causes lower test performance and is correlated with lower self-esteem and negative self-evaluations. Reducing test anxiety leads to improved test performance. A variety of interventions offer effective relief.

Kent, G., & Jambunathan, P. (1989). A longitudinal study of the intrusiveness of cognitions in test anxiety. *Behavior Research and Treatment, 27,* 43-50.

Changes over time in anxiety levels of 94 medical students were related to several parameters of intrusiveness, as well as to thought content.

Maultsby, M. (1975). *Help yourself to happiness.* New York: Institute of Rational Emotive Therapy.

Introduction to thought control for the general reader, like Ellis's books.

Russell, R. K., Wise, F., & Stratoudakis, J. P. (1976). Treatment of test anxiety by cue-controlled relaxation and systematic desensitization. *Journal of Counseling Psychology, 23,* 563-566.

Case study reports in which relaxation training reduced self-reported test anxiety.

Wine, J. D. (1980). Cognitive-attentional theory of test anxiety. In I. G. Sarason (Ed.), *Test anxiety, theory, research, and applications.* Hillsdale, NJ: Lawrence Erlbaum.

Cognitive coping skills training led to decreases in both state and trait measures of test anxiety and to increased performance on classroom tests.

Yerkes, R. M., & Dodson, J. D. (1908). The relation of strength of stimulus to rapidity of habit formation. *Journal of Comparative Neurology, 18,* 458-482.

Performance varies curvilinearly with motivation. Very low motivation leads to little effort and poor performance. Very high motivation can produce such tension that it interferes with performance. Moderate motivation results in optimal performance.

Fare Well!

We mean it. We hope this book helps you fare well in your studies. We believe the ideas we've presented will also be of assistance in your professional and personal lives. People who do what needs to be done on time, who have a knack for seeing the big picture while not forgetting the details, and who can stay reasonably calm and focused even in difficult situations are appreciated and respected by family, friends, and patients. If you start feeling disorganized or out of control as you continue your studies, please go back over the chapters of this book and remind yourself how to get back on track. Or for a different angle, read some of the references we've listed.

We'd love to hear from you! Let us know what has worked. Tell us if you've invented a new twist on any of our themes. We'd even like to see copies of your favorite charts, diagrams, or other notes that you found especially useful. You may write to us in care of the publisher or contact us directly at the e-mail address below:

> c/o Health Sciences Editor
> Sage Publications
> 2455 Teller Road
> Thousand Oaks, CA 91320
> e-mail: StudyWith@aol.com

We are also available to conduct Study Without Stress workshops for students and student-advising personnel. For more information you may contact us at the street or e-mail addresses above.

May your studies be without stress!

— Eugenia G. Kelman
— Kathleen C. Straker

Index

About the Authors

Eugenia G. Kelman, PhD, is a psychologist who has led test anxiety desensitization and general anxiety management groups at a university counseling center. She conducted research linking veterinary medical students' stress with fear of academic failure and discovered that students experiencing the most strain attributed their anxiety to lack of time, volume of information to learn, and consequent concern about testing. As assistant dean for student services, she designed academic support programs for veterinary medical students at Colorado State University and Cornell University. At the University of Texas Medical Branch, where she was Associate Director of the Counseling Center and Director of Academic Counseling Services, she conducted research concerning development of cognitive skills and developed academic enhancement programs, including study skills, time management, speed reading, and stress management.

Kathleen C. Straker is an educator and reading specialist who has worked in the Office of Student Affairs and the Office of Medical Education at the University of Texas Medical Branch. She served as Executive Chief Proctor for the National Board of Medical Examiners; codeveloped and coordinated the practical, clinical exercise for senior medical students; and worked extensively with the basic sciences faculty. She collaborated with Kelman in developing and offering study skills and reading enhancement workshops to medical students. She also has several years of teaching experience, having taught elementary through college classes. Currently, she works as a freelance writer in Houston, Texas.

Kelman and Straker offer workshops, based on their methodologies, to students and academic advisers.